Learning in the Workp...

This toolkit is designed to prepare health and social care practitioners for their role in facilitating learning in their workplace. It enables readers to recognise learning opportunities, communicate their professional knowledge, provide students with appropriate support, judge performance, coordinate student contact with others in the workplace and develop awareness of the needs of students from diverse backgrounds. It contains plenty of activities and questions, so that the reader can assess their knowledge base and apply the concepts in the toolkit to their work setting.

This new edition is fully updated and now includes international contexualisation, more coverage on meeting the diverse needs of students and a new section on meeting professional standards, which discusses the Nursing and Midwifery Council standards as well as those of other disciplines. A new companion website (www.routledge.com/cw/mulholland) makes valuable supplementary material available, including further activities and articles on managing the placement learning experience, developing new supervisors and making the most of reflection among others.

Practical and easy to read, this is an important resource for all those practitioners who support students in the workplace.

Joan Mulholland is Lecturer in the School of Nursing, University of Ulster, UK.

Chris Turnock is Academic Advisor, IT Services, Northumbria University, UK.

Learning in the Workplace

A toolkit for facilitating learning and assessment in health and social care settings

Second edition

Joan Mulholland and Chris Turnock

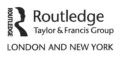

Routledge
Taylor & Francis Group

LONDON AND NEW YORK

First edition published 2007
by Kingsham Press

This edition published 2013
by Routledge
2 Park Square, Milton Park, Abingdon, Oxon, OX14 4RN

Simultaneously published in the USA and Canada
by Routledge
711 Third Avenue, New York, NY 10017

Routledge is an imprint of the Taylor & Francis Group, an informa business

British Library Cataloguing in Publication Data
A catalogue record for this book is available from the British Library

Library of Congress Cataloging-in-Publication Data
Mulholland, Joan, 1939–
Learning in the workplace : a toolkit for facilitating learning, and assessment in health, and
social care settings / Joan Mulholland and Chris Turnock. – 2nd ed.
p. cm.
Authors' names reversed on earlier ed.
Includes bibliographical references.
I. Turnock, Chris. II. Title.
[DNLM: 1. Allied Health Occupations–education. 2. Inservice Training–methods.
3. Learning. W 21.5]
LC classification not assigned
610.73'7069–dc23
2012012972

ISBN13: 978-0-415-53789-6 (hbk)
ISBN13: 978-0-415-53790-2 (pbk)
ISBN13: 978-0-203-10993-9 (ebk)

Typeset in Sabon by
FiSH Books Ltd, Enfield

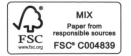

MIX
Paper from
responsible sources
FSC® C004839

Printed and bound in Great Britain by the MPG Books Group

Contents

Figures

Tables

Acknowledgements

The content of this toolkit has been based upon work that formed part of the Making Practice-Based Learning Work project. The Department of Employment and Learning (Northern Ireland) and the Higher Education Funding Council for England awarded a grant of £250,000 for the project, which involved collaboration between staff from Ulster, Northumbria and Bournemouth universities to make practitioners more effective in promoting the quality of practice-based learning. The project commenced in January 2003.

The project aimed to make practitioners more effective at supporting and supervising students in the workplace across a range of healthcare disciplines. The project undertook the following activities:

- Identifying and documenting good practice on preparing practitioners for their educational role.
- Developing and evaluating learning materials for practitioners.
- Disseminating learning materials across health and social care communities.

A number of key individuals were involved in the project's work, which culminated in production of learning materials and web-based resources that have formed the basis of this toolkit.

The authors would particularly like to thank Janet Scammell (Bournemouth University) for her input to all three phases of the project, Paula Moran (University of Ulster) for her input into Phases One and Two, Lynne Collier (Bournemouth University) for her input into Phase One and Tara Dixon (University of Ulster) for her input into Phase Three. We would also like thank Steve Mayman (Bournemouth University) for his input into production of the project's paper-based outputs and Julie Hunter and David Nichol (Northumbria University) for developing, updating and maintaining the project website.

In addition, the project website contains details of the various people who made a contribution to the project, but are too numerous to list here. Last but by no means least, our thanks go to Barbara Gregg for the administrative support she provided.

Finally, the authors would like to acknowledge Paula Moran's assistance in formulating many of the exercises used in this toolkit.

Joan Mulholland and Chris Turnock

Introduction

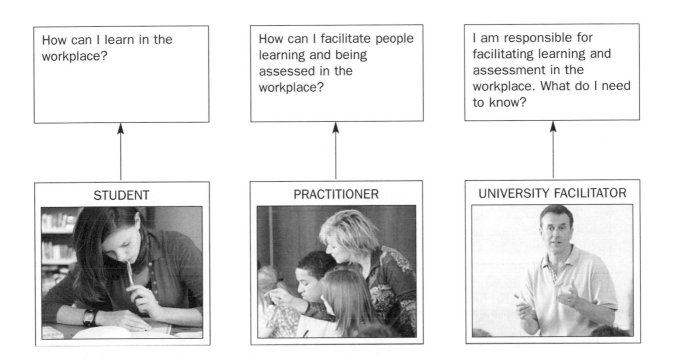

If you have asked yourself any of these questions, then this toolkit may help you answer them.

Many higher education courses require students to undergo a practice placement. Individuals responsible for facilitating learning and assessment in the workplace have been described in many ways. Table I.1 defines some of common titles in use and their associated roles.

Successful work-based learning needs facilitators who are able to recognise learning opportunities, communicate their professional knowledge, provide students with appropriate support, judge student performance, coordinate student contact with others in the workplace and have awareness of the needs of students from diverse backgrounds.

Courses in Health and Social Care that are accredited by statutory bodies do require that the work-based facilitator has met the required standards and competencies for their role. The General Social Care Council (2010), Health Professions Council (2009) and Nursing and Midwifery Council (2008) have all identified the standards that the facilitator is required to meet. The Higher Education Academy (2011), the Department of Health, Knowledge and Skills Framework (2004) and the Quality Assurance Agency for Higher Education (2006) also provide guidance and standards concerning work-based learning.

Table I.1 Common titles and roles

Title	Role description
Facilitator	Any individual supporting others to help bring about an outcome.
Mentor	A person who facilitates learning and supervises and assesses students in a practice setting.
Practice Educator	The role undertaken by health professionals supporting learning and assessment in practice.
Practice Supervisor	A person working with a student to manage the student's day-to-day activity and also contribute to the student's learning and assessment.
Practice Teacher	A person who has gained knowledge, skills and competence in both their specialist area of practice and in their teaching role, as well as in facilitating learning and supervising and assessing students.
Preceptor	Person providing support to others.
Sign-off Mentor	Mentors required to meet specified criteria in order to be able to sign off students' practice proficiency at the end of a practice placement.
Teacher	Someone who imparts knowledge.

The following list provides links to documents from a range of organisations and bodies that specifically relate to education and training standards:

- The NHS Knowledge and Skills Framework (NHS KSF) and the Development Review Process is available from the Department of Health website (use the 'search this site' facility for 'Knowledge and Skills Framework'): www.dh.gov.uk/en/Publicationsandstatistics/Publications/PublicationsPolicyAndGuidance/DH_4090843.
- Health Professions Council standards of education and training: www.hpc-uk.org/about registration/standards/sets/index.asp.
- This page on the Nursing and Midwifery Council's website provides access to the consultation document and final report of the 'Consultation on a Standard to Support Learning and Assessment in Practice': www.nmc-uk.org/Educators/Standards-for-education/Standards-to-support-learning-and-assessment-in-practice.
- The Chartered Society of Physiotherapy gives guidance to its Practice Educators via: www.csp.org.uk/professional-union/careers-development/practice-educators.
- The Accreditation of Practice Placement Educators (APPLE) scheme for Occupational Therapists has been developed primarily in order to give professional recognition to the role of the Practice Placement Educator (PPE): www.cot.co.uk/accreditation-practice-placement-educators-apple/accreditation-practice-placement-educators-apple.
- This Higher Education Authority site gives details of a 'Standards Framework for Teaching and Supporting Learning in Higher Education': www.heacademy.ac.uk/ukpsf.
- This page on the General Social Care Council's website gives access to quality assurance reports on social work education and the guidance document, 'Assessment of Practice in the Workplace': www.gscc.org.uk/page/126/Regulating+social+work+education.html.
- This is the Quality Assurance Agency for Higher Education's code of practice on assessing placement learning. It includes material on roles and responsibilities of the relevant parties in the assessment of practice-based learning: www.qaa.ac.uk/academicinfrastructure/codeOfPractice/section9/default.asp.

A consequence of these standards is that many practitioners need support to acquire the necessary knowledge and skills to provide effective support for a student undertaking a work-based placement. In addition, student supervision is often seen as an add-on activity as a result of insufficient numbers of suitably experienced and prepared staff, with such staff who are available being expected to cope with workloads that often fail to reflect their educational responsibilities (Spouse 2001).

The aim of this toolkit is to provide a potential facilitator with the material to prepare for the role of supporting a student undertaking a work-based placement. The toolkit may not only be useful to novice facilitators, but also more-experienced people who would like to enhance their role as a work-based facilitator. The toolkit has been designed so that the user can self-assess for a number of reasons. It enables the user to assess knowledge base, but also to apply the concepts in the toolkit to their work setting. The toolkit will also assist the work-based facilitator to meet relevant professional standards.

The Nursing and Midwifery Council's Standards to Support Learning and Assessment in Practice (2008) have identified eight domains that underpin this developmental framework. The eight domains in the framework identified outcomes at the four developmental stages. The domains are:

1 Establishing effective working relationships
2 Facilitation of learning
3 Assessment and accountability
4 Evaluation of learning
5 Creating an environment for learning
6 Context of practice
7 Evidence-based practice
8 Leadership

The toolkit has been mapped against these domains and will assist the practitioner in meeting the outcomes identified in the standards. Table I.2 (see pages 10–14) provides an example of how this toolkit might be used in relation to the eight domains.

An international perspective

Many other countries have also adopted a standards approach to the development of their health care facilitators and educators. The following organisations have identified standards that this toolkit can help facilitate the learner to meet.

Australia

- Nursing and midwifery: www.nursingmidwiferyboard.gov.au/Registration-Standards.aspx
- General practice nurses: www.anf.org.au/nurses_gp/index_rn.html
- Allied health professions, national standard for physiotherapists: www.physiocouncil.com.au/standards
- Paramedics (also covers New Zealand): www.paramedics.org.au/paramedics/competency-standards
- A state version that is more broad in nature: http://health.act.gov.au/professionals/allied-health/standards-of-practice

Canada

- Standards are produced on a state basis, and also by speciality for nursing
- There is a council of regulators, but at present very little about standards of professional practice on their web site: www.ccpnr.ca/index.html
- National standards for community nurses: www.chnc.ca/nursing-standards-of-practice.cfm

New Zealand

- Nursing: www.nursingcouncil.org.nz/index.cfm/1,40,0,0,html/Registered-Nurse
- Physiotherapy: www.physiotherapy.org.nz/Category?Action=View&Category_id=492

USA

- Nursing: www.nursingworld.org/nursingstandards
- Physiotherapy: https://www.fsbpt.org/ForCandidatesAndLicensees/ContinuingCompetence/Standards/index.asp
- Occupational therapists: www.aota.org/Practitioners/Licensure/StateRegs/ContComp.aspx

The toolkit contains exercises for users to explore ways to develop their own professional practice and also facilitate development of practice in the workplace. Each dimension of the assessment activity includes assessment of current practice in relation to a unit's topic, reflection and review of that practice, action planning to improve practice and, dependent on timescale, monitoring and review of the action plan. The material produced by undertaking these activities could be incorporated into a personal portfolio, which would contain evidence that users could present for formal academic accreditation with a higher education institution. Unit 7 provides guidance on completing a portfolio.

Many of these activities require consideration of the experience of supporting a student in the workplace. Readers with limited or no previous experience of student support should identify an experienced colleague and undertake a period of supervision before answering exercises relating to actual experience of supporting a student.

The toolkit uses the term facilitator to describe the person in the workplace who has been allocated to support an individual or group of students from a higher education institution undertaking a work-based placement. The toolkit also uses the terms, learner and student, to describe the student from a higher education institution or other organisation providing their education. These learners would normally be undertaking a work-based placement, though the toolkit recognises that this can include individuals who are learning in a workplace that is their normal place of work.

Learning outcomes of the toolkit

On completion of the toolkit you will have the following skills.

Knowledge and understanding of:

K1   the different ways people learn
K2   the range of methods used to aid learning in the workplace
K3   the roles and responsibilities of individuals associated with teaching and learning in the workplace
K4   different learning environments
K5   the need for assessment, the types of assessment in the workplace, and assessment and constructive feedback as an aid to learning
K6   the role of others and their contribution to learning in the workplace.

Intellectual qualities; the ability to:

I1   evaluate your role in providing support for learning
I2   investigate the need for assessment and use information from a range of disciplines
I3   apply theoretical concepts to teaching, learning and the assessment of students
I4   apply a critical approach to the collection, analysis and presentation of data.

Professional/practical skills; the ability to:

P1   develop the skills essential to successfully teach in the workplace
P2   design, plan, implement and evaluate a learning programme in the workplace
P3   demonstrate the skills required to effectively support learning in the workplace
P4   use a model of reflection to facilitate student learning in the workplace and facilitate a

process where the learner reflects critically on their practice

P5 demonstrate skills essential for effective assessment and identity strategies to manage failing students in the workplace

P6 plan, implement and evaluate assessment in the workplace

P7 develop a strategy for dealing with barriers in working with others, obtaining their cooperation and formulating and delivering effective methods of involving others to aid learning in the workplace.

Transferable skills; the ability to:

T1 discuss the use of reflection in learning and identify barriers to reflection and ways to minimise their effects

T2 facilitate a process where the learner reflects critically on their practice

T3 identify the diverse needs of individuals involved in learning and maximise individuals' potential for learning in the workplace

T4 work with a range of people from different backgrounds

T5 develop effective competencies as a placement teacher through the development of a portfolio of evidence

T6 evaluate your and your students' learning experience, reflect upon it and develop a personal development plan to further enhance this role.

Content

This toolkit contains seven units, each covering a main area of content which is further developed below. The units are:

1 Learning and teaching
2 Supporting learning in the workplace
3 Reflection on and in the workplace
4 Assessment in the workplace
5 Working with others in the workplace
6 Diversity
7 Portfolio completion guidelines.

Each unit is self-contained, but they build upon each other.

Teaching and learning methods

This toolkit is designed as an open-learning resource that provides users with the materials required to develop the skills, knowledge and attitudes for the facilitator role. These materials can be used independently, as part of a taught course or to enhance a claim for the Accreditation of Prior Experiential Learning. The toolkit may be used to inform a claim of meeting the Knowledge and Skills Framework (Department of Health 2004) or the professional or statutory body standards.

The toolkit contains practical exercises that bring theory and practice together, demonstrating their interrelationship and the underpinning concepts that inform how students are taught and assessed. The practical exercises will also assist in the development of a professional portfolio of evidence that can be submitted to an awarding authority for accreditation. Students will be directed to read and access materials from a wide range of sources. Students will be expected to engage with the materials and complete the exercises.

Assessment

The toolkit is not formally assessed, but may be submitted to your local higher education provider as an APEL claim against professional body and/or statutory body standards, for example Department of Health (2004), Health Professions Council (2009) and Nursing and Midwifery Council (2008).

As part of this assessment process you may be required to produce a portfolio of evidence; see Unit 7 for guidelines on completing a portfolio. Remember, the accrediting body and/or higher education provider will have specific requirements. We recommend that you find out what these requirements are before starting to produce your portfolio.

The units

The toolkit consists of seven units, each with a set of specific learning outcomes and content.

Unit 1: Learning and teaching in the workplace

Learning outcomes

On completing this unit, the facilitator will have:

- discussed the different ways in which people learn
- evaluated the range of methods used to aid learning in the workplace
- developed the skills essential to successfully teach in the workplace
- designed, planned, implemented and evaluated a learning programme in the workplace.

The content for the unit includes:

- theories of learning
- learning styles
- role of the teacher
- teaching methods and techniques
- skills in teaching in the workplace
- designing a learning programme.

Unit 2: Supporting learning in the workplace

Learning outcomes

On completing this unit, the facilitator will have:

- appraised the roles and responsibilities of individuals associated with teaching and learning in the workplace
- differentiated between different learning environments
- demonstrated the skills required to effectively support learning in the workplace
- evaluated his/her role in providing support for learning.

The content for the unit includes:

- discussion and definition of roles and responsibilities
- creation and maintenance of different learning environments to obtain different objectives
- resources available to support learning in the workplace
- development of skills essential to supporting learning and identifying learners' needs
- self-appraisal and continuing development in the individual's role as a learning supporter.

Unit 3: Reflection on and in the workplace

Learning outcomes

On completing this unit, the facilitator will have:

- discussed the use of reflection in learning
- identified barriers to reflection and ways to minimise their effects
- used a model of reflection to facilitate student learning in the workplace.

The content for the unit includes:

- what is reflective practice?
- becoming a reflective practitioner
- effective reflection supervision and assessment in the workplace
- learning through and from reflection
- reflection and evidence of competence
- mentoring and reflective practice
- learning from significant events
- reflective feedback
- tools for reflection.

Unit 4: Assessment in the workplace

Learning outcomes

On completing this unit, the facilitator will have:

- investigated the need for assessment
- analysed and compared the types of assessment in the workplace
- redefined assessment and constructive feedback as an aid to learning
- examined skills essential for effective assessment
- identified strategies to manage failing students in the workplace
- planned, implemented and evaluated assessment in the workplace.

The content for the unit includes:

- principles and needs of assessment
- different types of assessment
- suitable assessments in given situations
- giving constructive feedback
- developing and refining skills in constructive assessment
- the failing student
- availability of various resources to stimulate assessment sessions
- planning, implementation and evaluation to obtain a constructive assessment.

Unit 5: Working with others in the workplace

Learning outcomes

On completing this unit, the facilitator will have:

- recognised and understood the role of others and their contribution to learning in the workplace
- developed a strategy for dealing with barriers in working with others and obtaining their co-operation
- formulated and delivered effective methods for involving others to aid learning in the workplace.

The content for the unit includes:

- roles and responsibilities
- group dynamics
- groups and individuals
- individuals needs and difference
- assertiveness
- dealing with conflict
- communicating with others
- developing strategies for effective working.

Unit 6: Diversity in the workplace

Learning outcomes

On completing this unit, the facilitator will have:

- identified the diverse needs of individuals involved in learning
- maximised the individual's potential for learning in the workplace
- worked with a range of people from different backgrounds.

The content for the unit includes:

- nature of diversity
- ethnicity and culture
- religion and spirituality
- disability
- sexuality and gender
- age and generation
- class and socio-economic status
- strategies for working with people from diverse backgrounds.

Unit 7: Portfolio completion guidelines

Learning outcomes

On completing this unit, the facilitator will have:

- identified the requirements for completing a portfolio.

The content for the unit includes:

- preparing a portfolio
- submitting a portfolio
- portfolio assessment process.

Preparing for the toolkit

Please consider the following questions, as they will help prepare you for working through this toolkit. Write your responses in the spaces provided and return to them once you have worked through the units and reflect upon your original answers to see if you would answer the questions differently.

Context of learning in the workplace

1 What do you hope to gain from this toolkit?
2 List five words that describe how you would like to be viewed by students as a facilitator.
3 What do we mean when we say we are facilitating student learning in the workplace?
4 What is the value of reflection?
5 What are the characteristics of a good environment for learning in the workplace?
6 Why is assessment important in learning in the workplace?
7 How can you facilitate meeting the diverse needs of students who are learning in the workplace?

References

Department of Health (2004) *Knowledge and Skills Framework*. Department of Health.
General Social Care Council (2010) *Quality Assurance for Practice Learning*. www.gscc.org.uk/cmsFiles/Education%20and%20Training/QAPL_benchmark_statement_and_guidance_2nd_ed.pdf.
Health Professions Council (2009) *Standards of Education and Training*. Health Professions Council.
Higher Education Academy (2011) *The UK Professional Standards Framework*. www.heacademy.ac.uk/ukpsf.
Nursing and Midwifery Council (2008) *Standards to Support Learning and Assessing in Practice*. Nursing and Midwifery Council. www.nmc-uk.org/Documents/Standards/nmcStandardsToSupportLearning AndAssessmentInPractice.pdf.
Quality Assurance Agency for Higher Education (2006) *Code of Practice for the Assurance of Academic Quality and Standards in Higher Education: Placement Learning*. www.qaa.ac.uk/Publications/InformationAndGuidance/Documents/COP_AOS.pdf.
Spouse, J. (2001) Work-Based Learning in Health Care Environments. *Nurse Education in Practice* 1: 12–18.

Table I.2 Toolkit mapped against the eight developmental domains

NMC outcome	Learning resource/activity	Evidence that could go into your portfolio
Domain 1: *Establishing effective working relationships*		
Develop effective working relationships based on mutual trust and respect.	Read over existing orientation information for your ward or department.	Record in your portfolio a brief summary of this discussion highlighting key factors.
	Discuss with your supervisor factors that you consider to be important in promoting good working relationships.	
	Reflect on your experience of supporting students in practice; provide examples of factors that you consider to be important in promoting good working relationships.	
Demonstrate an understanding of factors that influence how students integrate into practice settings.	Unit 2: Supporting learning and teaching in the workplace • Roles and responsibilities	Include in portfolio a copy of your preparation plan.
	Construct a plan that demonstrates preparation for a student coming to your clinical area on placement.	Include a record of your discussion with your supervising mentor.
	Following commencement of this placement, evaluate how effective this was to help the student integrate into the practice setting.	
	Identify any changes that you might make in preparation for subsequent students. Discuss this with your supervising mentor.	
Provide on-going and constructive support to facilitate transition from one learning environment to another.	Unit 2: Supporting learning and teaching in the workplace • Learning environments • Mentoring	List the experiences that are available in your workplace for a student.
Domain 2: *Facilitation of learning*		
Use knowledge of the student's stage of learning to select appropriate learning opportunities to meet their individual needs.	Unit 1: Learning and teaching in the workplace • Learning contracts	Include a copy of the contract focusing on at least two of the students' learning outcomes.
	Construct a learning contract for a student on placement in your area based on the experiences available in your unit and link it to the student's learning outcomes.	

Facilitate selection of appropriate learning strategies to integrate learning from practice and academic experiences.	Unit 1: Learning and teaching in the workplace • Theories of learning • Learning styles • Assessing individual learning styles	Include in portfolio evidence of having completed the activity.
Support students in critically reflecting upon their learning experiences in order to enhance future learning.	Unit 3: Reflection in and on the workplace • Supervision	Complete activity 3.2 and include a brief synopsis of this in your portfolio.
Domain 3: Assessment and accountability		
Foster professional growth, personal development and accountability through support of students in practice.	Unit 2: Supporting learning and teaching in the workplace • Roles and responsibilities Discuss with a student their expectations of you as a mentor.	Write a description for your role as a mentor including key responsibilities and tasks.
Demonstrate a breadth of understanding of assessment strategies and the ability to contribute to the total assessment process as part of the teaching team.	Unit 4: Assessment in the workplace • Types of assessment	Select two course learning outcomes for a student in your clinical area and devise a plan showing how you think these could be assessed. Provide a rationale for your choice of assessment method.
Provide constructive feedback to students and assist them in identifying future learning needs and actions. Manage failing students so that they may either enhance their performance and capabilities for safe and effective practice or be able to understand their failure and the implications of this for their future.	Unit 4: Assessment in the workplace • Giving feedback • Helping a failing student Complete activities 4.7, 4.8 and 4.9 in Unit 4.	Summarise the ways in which you would support a student who is struggling in your area.
Be accountable for confirming that students have met, or not met, the NMC standards of proficiency in practice for registration – and at a level beyond initial registration – and are capable of safe and effective practice.	Unit 4: Assessment in the workplace • Skills for effective assessment • Student problems Undertake two assessments of practice under supervision.	Select one NMC Competency or Standard of Proficiency for a student in your area and specify the criteria you would use to confirm achievement or non-achievement using the following headings: Cognitive (knowledge) Psychomotor (doing) Affective (attitude).

Table 1.2 continued

NMC outcome	Learning resource/activity	Evidence that could go into your portfolio
Domain 4: Evaluation of learning		
Contribute to evaluation of student learning and assessment experiences, proposing aspects for change as a result of such evaluation.	Unit 4: Assessment in the workplace • Evaluating an assessment Complete a SWOT analysis on the learning environment in your workplace by using the form in Table 2.1, p. 68.	Identify the action you could take to improve the learning environment in your workplace.
Participate in self- and peer evaluation to facilitate personal development of others.	Unit 3: Reflection in and on the workplace • Keeping a reflective diary In discussion with your supervisor evaluate your performance in undertaking one student assessment by reflecting on your strengths and areas that require further developments. Record a summary of this.	Include a copy of your summary evaluation.
Domain 5: Creating an environment for learning		
Support students to identify both learning needs and experiences that are appropriate to their level of training.	Unit 2: Supporting learning and teaching in the workplace • Learning environments Locate in the appropriate curriculum document the learning outcomes a student should achieve as a result of being on a clinical placement with you. In conjunction with a student, design a learning contract to reflect these learning outcomes and the student's expectations of the placement.	Learning contract.
Use a range of learning experiences, involving patients, clients, carers and the professional team, to meet defined learning needs.	Unit 2: Supporting learning and teaching in the workplace • Learning environments Using the above learning contract, discuss with your supervisor the resources/experiences available to meet the stated learning outcomes.	List of identified resources.

Identify aspects of the learning environment that could be enhanced – negotiating with others to make appropriate changes.	Unit 2: Supporting learning and teaching in the workplace • Learning environments Complete a SWOT analysis of the learning environment in your workplace by using the form in Table 2.1, p. 68. Select one of the opportunities that you have identified and discuss with your supervising mentor how this could be utilised to enhance students' learning.	SWOT analysis. Outline the main parts of this discussion in your portfolio.
Act as a resource to facilitate personal and professional development of others.	Unit 6: Diversity in the workplace • Strategies for supporting all students Review the learning contract already compiled. Select a learning opportunity. Prepare and deliver a teaching session. Reflect on your teaching practice and your one-to-one contact with the student, using the headings below; in what way do you think you could improve your communication skills? Discuss with your supervisor.	Briefly outline how you could incorporate these developments into your work with students.

Domain 6: Context of practice

Contribute to the development of an environment in which effective practice is fostered, implemented, evaluated and disseminated.	Using the HEI & DHSSPSNI Educational Audit tool, complete an educational audit for the clinical facility that you are working in and compare to the existing document held in the ward.	Copy of the audit tool that you have completed of your audit of the clinical area.
Set and maintain professional boundaries that are sufficiently flexible for providing inter-professional care.	Design an activity to assist the student in being able to identify the roles and responsibilities of an individual or group in the workplace and their importance to the learning experience. Evaluate and reflect upon the effectiveness of the activity and make recommendations for its development.	Record a brief outline of the evaluation and recommendations.
Initiate and respond to practice developments to ensure that safe and effective care is achieved and an effective learning environment is maintained.	Access on the RQIA website a recent report and consider how the recommendations for practice development are being implemented into current practice. http://www.rqia.org.uk.	Provide evidence to demonstrate how practice in your area has responded to the identified recommendation.

Table I.2 continued

NMC outcome	Learning resource/activity	Evidence that could go into your portfolio
Domain 7: Evidence-based practice		
Identify and apply research and evidence-based practice to their area of practice.	Make a list of 3 aspects of your clinical work where you can immediately relate to an available evidence base (current research).	Outline what strategies are in place in your area to ensure practice is evidence based.
Contribute to strategies to increase or review the evidence base used to support practice.	Use this information when working with a student to review available or new evidence in regard to a particular practice in your clinical environment.	
Support students in applying an evidence base to their own practice.	Review with a student the definitions of the following key terms: • Evidence-based practice • Clinical effectiveness and audit • Research and development • Practice development. Plan a learning activity in your environment that will allow you to assess your students' understanding of the key terms above. Include a copy of the learning activity in your portfolio.	
Domain 8: Leadership		
Plan a series of learning experiences that will meet students' defined learning needs.	Review the learning contract already compiled. Prepare and deliver teaching session(s) to meet student learning needs.	Evidence already captured in portfolio.
Be an advocate for students to support them in accessing learning opportunities that meet their individual needs – involving a range of other professionals, patients, clients and carers.	Unit 5: Working with others in the workplace • Individuals' needs and differences Discuss with your supervisor your thoughts on how individuals and groups work effectively.	Include a summary from your discussion.
Prioritise work to accommodate support of students within their practice roles.	Reflect on the responsibilities of your role as a practitioner and a mentor. Identify areas of possible conflict or difficulty. Discuss these with both your line manager and supervisor.	Outline a plan to overcome any difficulties identified.
Provide feedback about the effectiveness of learning and assessment in practice.	Discuss the effectiveness of learning and assessment in practice with your supervisor and, if possible, link lecturer.	Include a copy of anonymized student assessment documentation in your portfolio. Include a summary from your discussion.

Learning and teaching in the workplace

Introduction

The work-based facilitator requires an understanding of the principles of learning theory and their application to teaching in the workplace. The ability to use research to both inform teaching methods and content of practice-based education is fundamental to good teaching practice. This section will explore the ways in which people learn, including their learning styles and the role of the teacher in facilitating learning in the workplace. The section also examines various teaching methods that can be used in workplace learning as well as dealing with difficult situations and designing a learning programme.

Aim of the unit

The aim of this unit is to examine the way in which adults learn and to consider the skills required for effective teaching.

Outcomes of the unit

At the end of this unit you will be able to:

1   discuss the different ways that people learn
2   evaluate the range of methods used to aid learning in the workplace
3   develop the skills essential to successfully teach in the workplace
4   design, plan, implement and evaluate a learning programme in the workplace.

ACTIVITY 1.1

The following exercise is designed to help you to understand how you are assisted to learn and to identify different theories of learning.

You are undertaking a university course and notice that the lecturers use different approaches. When you ask why, you are told that they use different theories of learning. Read the following section and answer these questions:

* Which of the theories helps you learn most?
* Which theory do you learn least from?

Theories of learning

There are various theories of learning. One website (Kearsley 2012) lists over 50 different theories. This unit will provide you with an overview of a selection of mainstream theories that are particularly pertinent to the role of the work-based facilitator.

Andragogy

Knowle's theory of andragogy (Knowles 1975, 1984) is an attempt to develop a theory specifically for adult learning. Knowles emphasises that adults are self-directed and expect to take responsibility for decisions. Adult-learning programmes must accommodate this fundamental aspect.

Andragogy makes the following assumptions about the design of learning: (1) adults need to know why they need to learn something; (2) adults need to learn experientially; (3) adults approach learning as problem-solving; and (4) adults learn best when the topic is of immediate value.

In practical terms, andragogy means that instruction for adults needs to focus more on the process and less on the content being taught. Strategies such as case studies, role-playing, simulations and self-evaluation are most useful. Instructors adopt a role of facilitator or resource, rather than lecturer or grader.

Andragogy applies to any form of adult learning and has been used extensively in the design of organisational training programmes (especially for 'soft skill' domains such as management development).

Principles of andragogy

1 Adults need to be involved in the planning and evaluation of their instruction.
2 Experience (including mistakes) provides the basis for learning activities.
3 Adults are most interested in learning subjects that have immediate relevance to their job or personal life.
4 Adult learning is problem-centred rather than content-oriented.

Constructivist theory

A major theme in the theoretical framework of Bruner is that learning is an active process in which learners construct new ideas or concepts based upon their current/past knowledge. The learner selects and transforms information, constructs hypotheses and makes decisions, relying on a cognitive structure, i.e. a mental model, to do so. Cognitive structure provides meaning and organisation to experiences and allows the individual to 'go beyond the information given'.

As far as instruction is concerned, the instructor should try and encourage students to discover principles by themselves. The instructor and student should engage in an active dialogue (i.e. Socratic learning). The task of the instructor is to translate information to be learned into a format appropriate to the learner's current state of understanding. Curriculum should be organised in a spiral manner, so that the student continually builds upon what they have already learned.

Bruner (1966) states that instruction should address four major aspects: (1) predisposition towards learning; (2) the ways in which a body of knowledge can be structured so that it can be most readily grasped by the learner; (3) the most effective sequences in which to present material; and (4) the nature and pacing of rewards and punishments. Good methods for structuring knowledge should result in simplifying, generating new propositions and increasing the manipulation of information.

Bruner's constructivist theory is a general framework for instruction based upon the study of cognition. Much of the theory is linked to child development research (especially Piaget). The ideas outlined in Bruner (1960) originated from a conference focused on science and maths learning. Bruner illustrated his theory in the context of mathematics and social science programmes for young children (see Bruner 1973). Note that constructivism is a very broad conceptual framework in philosophy and science and Bruner's theory represents one particular perspective.

Principles of constructivist theory

1 Instruction must be concerned with the experiences and contexts that make the student willing and able to learn (readiness).
2 Instruction must be structured so that it can be easily grasped by the student (spiral organisation).
3 Instruction should be designed to facilitate extrapolation and/or fill in the gaps (going beyond the information given).

Experiential learning – Kolb

The core of Kolb's four-stage model (Kolb 1984) is a simple description of the learning cycle which shows how experience is translated through reflection into concepts, which in turn are used as guides for active experimentation and the choice of new experiences. Kolb refers to these four stages as: *concrete experience* (CE), *reflective observation* (RO), *abstract conceptualisation* (AC) and *active experimentation* (AE). They follow each other in a cycle, which may be entered at any point, but the stages should be followed in sequence (see Figure 1.1).

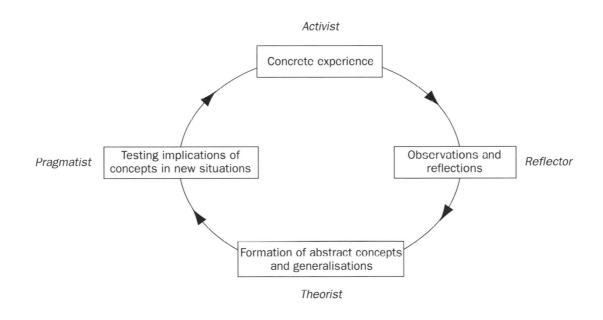

Figure 1.1 The Lewinian experiential learning model (after Kolb 1984, p. 21)

Each of the four stages of the cycle involves:

- planning and preparing
- identifying a gap between our present state and our desired state, representing a need
- planning some activity and identifying the resources required to meet that need
- specifying the criteria and evidence that will let us know it is being met
- action
- engaging in the activity

- reflection
- reflecting on that experience and gathering information
- concluding
- beginning to generalise and internalise what happened with that experience.

Comparing our present state and desired state using the evidential criteria, and using these conclusions to carry on to a further stage of preparing and planning, the learning cycle thus provides feedback, which is the basis for new action and evaluation of the consequences of that action. Learners should go through the cycle several times, so it may best be thought of as a spiral of cycles. In brief, Kolb conceptualises the process of action research as a spiral of action and research consisting of four major moments: *plan, act, observe* and *reflect*.

Principles of experiential learning – Kolb

What is important is to systematically take the learner around each stage of the cycle, ensuring that effective links are made between each stage. The model offers an explicit critique of those highly theoretical programmes or courses that do not value the prior experience or knowledge of students. It is similarly critical of those experiential activities (for example, certain field courses, simulations and games) where students receive little preparation for the experience and/or no effective chance to reflect upon the experience and relate it to their wider reading or the more explicitly theoretical aspects of the course.

Experiential learning – Rogers

Rogers (1969) distinguished two types of learning: cognitive (meaningless) and experiential (significant). The former corresponds to academic knowledge such as learning vocabulary or multiplication tables and the latter refers to applied knowledge such as learning about engines in order to repair a car. The key to the distinction is that experiential learning addresses the needs and wants of the learner. Rogers lists these qualities of experiential learning: personal involvement, self-initiated, evaluated by learner and pervasive effects on learner.

To Rogers, experiential learning is equivalent to personal change and growth. Rogers feels that all human beings have a natural propensity to learn; the role of the teacher is to facilitate such learning. This includes: (1) setting a positive climate for learning; (2) clarifying the purposes of the learner(s); (3) organising and making available learning resources; (4) balancing intellectual and emotional components of learning; and (5) sharing feelings and thoughts with learners, but not dominating.

According to Rogers, learning is facilitated when: (1) the student participates completely in the learning process and has control over its nature and direction; (2) it is primarily based upon direct confrontation with practical, social, personal or research problems; and (3) self-evaluation is the principal method of assessing progress or success. Rogers also emphasises the importance of learning to learn and an openness to change.

Roger's theory of learning originates from his views about psychotherapy and humanistic approach to psychology. It applies primarily to adult learners and has influenced other theories of adult learning such as adult learning theory and andragogy. Combs (1982) considers the significance of Roger's work to education. Rogers and Freiberg (1994) discuss applications of the experiential learning framework to the classroom.

Principles of experiential learning – Rogers

1   Significant learning takes place when the subject matter is relevant to the personal interests of the student.
2   Learning that is threatening to the self (e.g. new attitudes or perspectives) is more easily assimilated when external threats are at a minimum.
3   Learning proceeds faster when the threat to the self is low.
4   Self-initiated learning is the most lasting and pervasive.

Operant conditioning

The theory of B.F. Skinner (Skinner 1953) is based upon the idea that learning is a function of change in overt behaviour. Changes in behaviour are the result of an individual's response to events (stimuli) that occur in the environment. A response produces a consequence such as defining a word, hitting a ball, or solving a maths problem. When a particular Stimulus-Response (S-R) pattern is reinforced (rewarded), the individual is conditioned to respond. The distinctive characteristic of operant conditioning relative to previous forms of behaviourism is that the organism can emit responses instead of only eliciting response due to an external stimulus.

Reinforcement is the key element in Skinner's S-R theory. A reinforcer is anything that strengthens the desired response. It could be verbal praise, a good grade or a feeling of increased accomplishment or satisfaction. The theory also covers negative reinforcers, i.e. any stimulus that results in the increased frequency of a response when it is withdrawn (different from aversive stimuli, namely punishment, which result in reduced responses). A great deal of attention was given to schedules of reinforcement (e.g. interval versus ratio) and their effects on establishing and maintaining behaviour.

One of the distinctive aspects of Skinner's theory is that it attempted to provide behavioural explanations for a broad range of cognitive phenomena. For example, Skinner explained drive (motivation) in terms of deprivation and reinforcement schedules. Skinner (1957) tried to account for verbal learning and language within the operant conditioning paradigm, although this effort was strongly rejected by linguists and psycholinguists. Skinner (1988) deals with the issue of free will and social control.

Operant conditioning has been widely applied in clinical settings (i.e. behaviour modification) as well as teaching (i.e. classroom management) and instructional development (e.g. programmed instruction). Paradoxically, it should be noted that Skinner rejected the idea of theories of learning; see Skinner (1950) for more information.

Principles of operant conditioning

1 Behaviour that is positively reinforced will reoccur; intermittent reinforcement is particularly effective.
2 Information should be presented in small amounts so that responses can be reinforced ('shaping').
3 Reinforcements will generalise across similar stimuli ('stimulus generalisation') producing secondary conditioning.

Social learning theory

The social learning theory of Bandura emphasises the importance of observing and modelling the behaviours, attitudes, and emotional reactions of others. Bandura (1977) states that learning would be exceedingly laborious, not to mention hazardous, if people had to rely solely on the effects of their own actions to inform them what to do. Fortunately, most human behaviour is learned observationally through modelling: from observing others one forms an idea of how new behaviours are performed, and on later occasions this coded information serves as a guide for action.

Social learning theory explains human behaviour in terms of continuous reciprocal interaction between cognitive, behavioural and environmental influences. The component processes underlying observational learning are: attention, retention, motor reproduction and motivation.

Because it encompasses attention, memory and motivation, social learning theory spans both cognitive and behavioural frameworks. Bandura's work is related to the theories that also emphasise the central role of social learning.

Social learning theory has been applied extensively to the understanding of aggression (Bandura 1973) and psychological disorders, particularly in the context of behaviour modification (Bandura 1969). It is also the theoretical foundation for the technique of behaviour modelling that is widely used in training programmes. In recent years, Bandura has focused his work on the concept of self-efficacy in a variety of contexts (e.g. Bandura 1997).

Principles of social learning theory

1 The highest level of observational learning is achieved by first organising and rehearsing the modelled behaviour symbolically and then enacting it overtly. Coding modelled behaviour into words, labels or images results in better retention than simply observing.
2 Individuals are more likely to adopt a modelled behaviour if it results in outcomes that they value.
3 Individuals are more likely to adopt a modelled behaviour if the model is similar to the observer and has admired status and the behaviour has functional value.

Structural learning

According to structural learning theory (Scandura 2012), one learns rules that consist of a domain, range and procedure. There may be alternative rule sets for any given class of tasks. Problem-solving may be facilitated when higher order rules are used, i.e. rules that generate new rules. Higher order rules account for creative behaviour (unanticipated outcomes) as well as the ability to solve complex problems by making it possible to generate (learn) new rules.

Structural analysis is a methodology for identifying the rules to be learned for a given topic or class of tasks and breaking them done into their atomic components. The major steps in structural analysis re: (1) select a representative sample of problems; (2) identify a solution rule for each problem; (3) convert each solution rule into a higher-order problem whose solution is that rule; (4) identify a higher-order solution rule for solving the new problems; (5) eliminate redundant solution rules from the rule set (i.e. those that can be derived from other rules); and (6) notice that steps 3 and 4 are essentially the same as steps 1 and 2, and continue the process iteratively with each newly identified set of solution rules. The result of repeatedly identifying higher-order rules, and eliminating redundant rules, is a succession of rule sets, each consisting of rules that are simpler individually but collectively more powerful than the ones before.

Structural learning describes teaching as first seeking the simplest solution path for a problem and then teaching more complex paths until the entire rule has been mastered. The theory proposes that we should teach as many higher-order rules as possible as replacements for lower-order rules. The theory also suggests a strategy for individualising instruction by analysing which rules a student has/has not mastered and teaching only the rules, or portions thereof, that have not been mastered.

Principles of structural learning

1 Whenever possible, teach higher-order rules that can be used to derive lower-order rules.
2 Teach the simplest solution path first and then teach more complex paths or rule sets.
3 Rules must be composed of the minimum capabilities possessed by the learners.

Constructive alignment

The model below, adapted from Biggs (2011), describes four levels of thinking about learning and teaching. The levels, range from Level One, where the student is merely a 'sponge' absorbing material without too much thought as to where the knowledge is taking them, to Level Four, where the student is actively engaged in management of their own learning. In this model, levels of thinking about learning are defined in terms of what is focused upon, i.e. what the student does as a response to teaching.

Level One: The focus is on what the student is: '*A teacher's responsibility is to know the content well and to expound it clearly. Thereafter, it's up to the students. When students don't learn . . . it is due to something the students are lacking.*'

Level Two: The focus is on what the teacher does. '*The teacher who operates at level 2 works at obtaining an armoury of teaching skills.*' However, '*Level 2 is also a defect model, the "blame" this time being on the teacher.*' Biggs argues, '*The focus should not be on the skills itself, but whether its deployment has the desired effect on student learning*' and goes on to describe a desirable third level.

Level Three: The focus is on what the student does. '*Level 3 sees teaching as support learning.*' It recognises that learning can only be effective if it is engaged in actively by the learner, and the teacher's task, which may involve the deployment of a great many Level Two skills, is to set up an environment of learning activities and assessment from which it is very difficult for the student to escape without learning.

Level Four: The focus is on how the student can manage what they do, initially within frameworks created by the teacher, but ultimately negotiating or creating his or her own framework. This level links to Personal Development Planning and the idea of the independent learner. There is no short cut from Levels One or Two straight to Level Four. A student cannot operate effectively at Level Four without having experienced Level Three teaching of constructive alignment.

Principles of constructive alignment

1 Students construct meaning from what they do to learn.
2 The teacher aligns the planned learning activities with the learning outcomes.

Deep and surface learning

Finally, one perspective upon learning theory identifies two types of learning, deep and surface learning. Deep learning involves the critical analysis of new ideas, linking them to already known concepts and principles, and leads to understanding and long-term retention of concepts so that they can be used for problem-solving in unfamiliar contexts. Deep learning promotes understanding and application for life.

In contrast, surface learning is the tacit acceptance of information and memorisation as isolated and unlinked facts. It leads to superficial retention of material for examinations and does not promote understanding or long-term retention of knowledge and information.

Table 1.1 compiled from the work of Entwistle (1988), Ramsden (2003) and Biggs (2011) provides some very valuable characteristics of the two approaches and illustrates the importance of how teaching impacts on the learning process.

Principles of deep learning

The last row of the table provides us with some simple guidelines as to the 'do's' and 'don'ts' in teaching. In order to encourage active learning, teachers need to concentrate on the key concepts, not just in isolation, but also by demonstrating the way that the components link together. Over-reliance on traditional lectures, where students are passively taking notes and not being required to engage actively with material, will not encourage a deep approach. Similarly, over-assessment, through repeated testing, while being seen to regularly focus the learners on the material, is likely to have the opposite effect to that desired by just encouraging the memorising of facts.

Critical to our understanding of this principle is that we should not identify the student with a fixed approach to learning, but design learning opportunities that encourage students to adopt a particular approach. This work indicates the need to understand both the different styles of learning and approaches to teaching so that the work-based facilitator can utilise strategies for effective student teaching.

ACTIVITY 1.2

Having considered the various theoretical models of learning and teaching, answer the following question.

You have been asked to teach a practical skill to a student. Which two learning theories would be best for teaching this skill in your workplace?

Table 1.1 Characteristics and factors that encourage deep and surface approaches to learning

	Deep learning	Surface learning
Definition	Examining new facts and ideas critically, tying them into existing cognitive structures and making numerous links between ideas.	Accepting new facts and ideas uncritically and attempting to store them as isolated, unconnected items.
Characteristics	Looking for meaning.	Relying on rote learning.
	Focussing on the central argument or *concepts* needed to solve a problem.	Focussing on outwards signs and the *formulae* needed to solve a problem.
	Interacting actively.	Receiving information passively. Failing to distinguish principles from examples.
	Distinguishing between argument and evidence.	
	Making connections between different modules.	Treating parts of modules and programmes as separate.
	Relating new and previous knowledge.	Not recognising new material as building on previous work.
	Linking course content to real life.	Seeing course content simply as material to be learnt for the exam.
Encouraged by students'	Having an intrinsic curiosity in the subject.	Studying a degree for the qualification and not being interested in the subject.
	Being determined to do well and mentally engaging when doing academic work.	Not focussing on academic areas, but emphasising others (e.g. social, sporting).
	Having the appropriate background knowledge for a sound foundation.	Lacking background knowledge and understanding necessary to understand material.
	Having time to pursue interests, through good time management.	Not enough time/too high a workload.
	Positive experience of education leading to confidence in ability to understand and succeed.	Cynical view of education, believing that factual recall is what is required.
		High anxiety.
Encouraged by teachers'	Showing personal interest in the subject.	Conveying disinterest or even a negative attitude to the material.
	Bringing out the structure of the subject.	Presenting material so that it can be perceived as a series of unrelated facts and ideas.
	Concentrating on and ensuring plenty of time for key concepts.	Allowing students to be passive.
	Confronting students' misconceptions.	Assessing for independent facts (short-answer questions).
	Engaging students in active learning.	
	Using assessments that require thought, and require ideas to be used together.	Rushing to cover too much material.
	Relating new material to what students already know and understand.	Emphasising coverage at the expense of depth.
	Allowing students to make mistakes without penalty and rewarding effort.	Creating undue anxiety or low expectations of success by discouraging statements or by excessive workload.
	Being consistent and fair in assessing declared intended learning outcomes, and hence establishing trust.	Having a short assessment cycle.

Source: Compiled from Entwistle (1988), Ramsden (1992) and Biggs (1999)

Summary

It is important to note that there is no single theory that can be applied to all adults or learning situations. Instead, you need to use the principles of various theories, depending on the learner as well as the nature of the learning that needs to take place.

Learning styles

Introduction

The basic principle behind the theory of learning styles is that different people learn in different ways. There is much literature on learning styles and, as with much educational theory, there are some differences of opinion particularly in classification of the different styles.

ACTIVITY 1.3

In light of the statement in the paragraph above, namely that people learn in different ways, think about how you learn best.

Which of the following do you learn by?

- doing an activity
- reading about a topic
- reflecting on your experiences
- working with others
- watching a video.

Now read the following section on learning styles to help you understand more about your preferred learning style.

Kolb (1984) suggests that students develop a preference for learning in a particular way. The preferred style reflects a tendency rather than an absolute, and students may adopt different learning styles in different situations, but they tend to favour some learning behaviours in preference to others. He identifies four learning styles, each of which is associated with a different way of solving problems:

1 *Divergers* – view situations from many perspectives and rely heavily upon brainstorming and generation of ideas.
2 *Assimilators* – use inductive reasoning and have the ability to create theoretical models.
3 *Convergers* – rely heavily on hypothetical-deductive reasoning.
4 *Accommodators* – carry out plans and experiments and adapt to immediate circumstances.

Another model (Felder 1993) identifies four learning style dimensions.

1 Active-reflective dimension
   - Active learners:
     - retain and understand information best by discussing it, applying it or explaining it to others
     - 'let's try it out and see how it works'
     - prefer group work
     - find it difficult to sit in lectures just taking notes; require interaction.
   - Reflective learners:
     - retain and understand information best by thinking about it first
     - 'let's think it through first'
     - prefer working alone
     - need thinking time during lectures.

2   Sensing-intuitive dimension
  • Sensing learners:
    ○ like to learn facts
    ○ like to solve problems using well-established methods and dislike complications and surprises
    ○ tend to be patient with details and are good at memorising facts and doing hands-on work, e.g. labs and projects
    ○ tend to be more practical and careful
    ○ do not like courses that have no apparent connection to the real world
  • Intuitive learners:
    ○ prefer discovering possibilities and relationships
    ○ like innovation and dislike repetition
    ○ may be better at grasping new concepts and are more comfortable with abstract material and mathematical formulations
    ○ tend to work faster and are more innovative, but may be careless
    ○ do not like courses that involve a lot of memorisation and routine calculations.
3   Visual-verbal dimension
  • Visual learners:
    ○ remember best what they see, e.g. pictures, diagrams, demonstrations
  • Verbal learners:
    ○ get more out of words, whether written or spoken explanations.
4   Sequential-global dimension
  • Sequential learners:
    ○ gain understanding in small, sequential, logical steps
    ○ tend to follow logical (stepwise) paths while problem-solving
    ○ may not understand material fully but are still able to solve problems and pass tests
    ○ may know a lot about specific aspects of a subject, but may have trouble relating them to different aspects of the same or different subjects.
  • Global learners:
    ○ seem to learn in large jumps, absorbing material almost randomly without seeing connections, then suddenly 'getting it'
    ○ may be able to solve complex problems quickly, or put things together in a novel way once they have grasped the big picture
    ○ may have severe difficulties in solving problems when they have not grasped everything (strongly global learners)
    ○ may have difficulty in explaining their knowledge.

Felder and Silverman (1998) developed a model of student preferences in their learning:

• What type of information does the student preferentially perceive: sensory (external) – sights, sounds, physical sensations; or intuitive (internal) – possibilities, insights, hunches?
• Through which sensory channel is external information most effectively perceived: visual – pictures, diagrams, graphs, demonstrations; or auditory – words, sounds?
• How does the student prefer to process information: actively – through engagement in physical activity or discussion; or reflectively – through introspection?
• How does the student progress toward understanding: sequentially – in continual steps; or globally – in large jumps, holistically?

A number of cognitive styles have been identified and studied over the years. Field independence versus field dependence is probably the most well-known style. This refers to a tendency to approach the environment in an analytical, as opposed to global, fashion. At a perceptual level, field independent personalities are able to distinguish figures as discrete from their backgrounds compared to field dependent individuals who experience events in an undifferentiated way. In addition, field dependent individuals have a greater social orientation relative to field independent personalities. Studies have identified a number of connections between this cognitive style and learning, see Messick (1978). For example, field independent individuals are likely to learn more effectively under conditions of intrinsic motivation (e.g. self-study) and are influenced less by social reinforcement.

Hibernia College (2012) identifies various learning styles, as described below.

Visual

These learners need to see the teacher's body language and facial expression to fully understand the content of a lesson. They tend to prefer sitting at the front of the classroom to avoid visual obstructions (e.g. people's heads). They may think in pictures and learn best from visual displays including: diagrams, illustrated text books, overhead transparencies, videos, flipcharts and hand-outs. During a lecture or classroom discussion, visual learners often prefer to take detailed notes to absorb the information.

People who have a visual learning style learn best if a major component of the material or lesson is something they can see or watch. This learner works best with written material and instructions, diagrams, posters and demonstrations. The information which the visual learner takes in is translated into and stored as pictures or images in their brains. These learners are usually neat and well organised. They may use statements with visual cues such as 'I get the picture'. Unnecessary movement can be a distraction to a visual learner.

Careers that suit the visual learner would include executive positions where a vision of the future is important, architects, engineers and surgeons.

Auditory

Auditory learners interpret the underlying meanings of speech through listening to tone of voice, pitch, speed and other nuances. Written information may have little meaning until it is heard. These learners often benefit from reading text aloud and using a tape recorder.

People who have an auditory learning style learn best if there is an oral component to the material being learned. Verbal instructions, taped lectures and face-to-face instruction work best. These learners filter the information they hear and store the relevant data but don't necessarily form pictures around it. Auditory learners prefer to 'talk it out' when problem-solving. While talking they may use phrases which relate to how they learn such as, 'I hear you'. Unnecessary noise can be a distraction for the auditory learner.

Because of their excellent listening skills, auditory learners would make excellent pathologists, disc jockeys, and musicians.

Kinesthetic

Tactile/kinesthetic persons learn best through a hands-on approach, actively exploring the physical world around them. They may find it hard to sit still for long periods and may become distracted by their need for activity and exploration.

People who have a kinesthetic or tactile learning style learn best when they can touch or feel what they are learning about. The use of their body and feelings are very important to these learners so hands-on projects work best for them. Kinesthetic learners do not always have a good time sense or sense of orderliness or neatness. They often live for the moment and do not have a vision of the future. Kinesthetic learners will often speak of their learning in terms of feelings, prefacing statements with 'I feel'. People with this learning style will have a tendency to move around while trying to solve a problem.

Career choices for people with this learning style should be anything that involves movement and their body, such as dancing, acting, construction or athletics.

ACTIVITY 1.4

The following activity asks you to consider how you learn and how this may apply to your teaching.

Reflect on your own learning style using the links in the following section on assessing individual learning styles.

What are the strengths and weaknesses of your learning style?

How does your learning style impact on how you teach students?

Can you think of aspects of your teaching that you would want to develop?

How could you further develop these aspects? (This may be useful to include in your portfolio.)

Assessing individual learning styles

The particular choice of learning style reflects the individual's abilities, environment and learning history (Nulty and Barrett 1996). According to Kolb (1984), learners learn better when the subject matter is presented in a style consistent with their preferred learning style.

There are a number of tools to assess learning style, for example:

- http://members.shaw.ca/mdde615/lrnstylsquiz7.htm
- www.advisorteam.com/temperament_sorter/register.asp?partid=1
- www.ldpride.net/learning_style.html

Left to their own devices, students tend to do what is easiest for them, which is to use their own learning style. Similarly, individual teachers may teach in ways that reflect their own learning styles and implicitly assume that all their students learn that way. However, there is evidence that learning (or at least retention) is enhanced as more of the learning stages are used (Felder and Brent 2005). This confirms Kolb's argument that teachers need to encourage students to engage with all four stages of the learning cycle.

Students should not be labelled as having one fixed learning style; instead, work-based facilitators need to recognise that individuals will have particular modes of learning that are more dominant than others. Facilitators need to adopt approaches to teaching that enable students who have different learning styles to learn effectively. This means that the role of the teacher includes designing learning opportunities to ensure that work-based learning is accessible to the largest number of students.

Role of the teacher

Kearsley (2012) outlines various aspects of the teacher role, which can be utilised for teaching in the workplace.

Feedback

Feedback and reinforcement are two of the most pivotal concepts in learning. Feedback involves providing learners with information about their responses, whereas reinforcement affects the tendency to make a specific response again. Feedback can be positive, negative or neutral; reinforcement is either positive (increases the response) or negative (decreases the response). Feedback is almost always considered external, while reinforcement can be external or intrinsic (i.e. generated by the individual).

The nature of the feedback or reinforcement provided was the basis for many early instructional principles. For example, the use of 'prompting' (i.e. providing hints) was recommended in order to 'shape' (i.e. selectively reinforce) the correct responses. Other principles concerned the choice of an appropriate 'step size' (i.e. how much information to present at once) and how often feedback or reinforcement should be provided.

Daloz's (1986) two-level feedback model identifies support and challenge as fundamental aspects of feedback. The best feedback is high on support and high on challenge (see Figure 1.2).

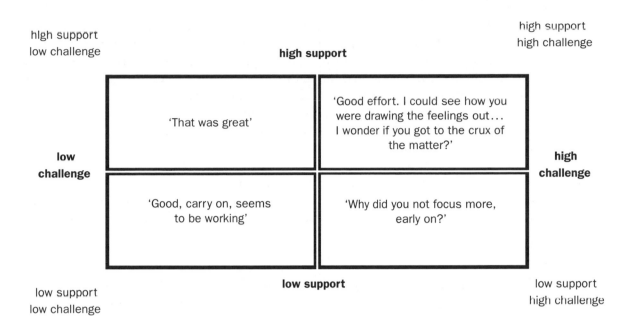

Figure 1.2 Daloz (1986) feedback model

The important thing is to make sure that the feedback is both timely and constructive. Some guiding principles are to:

- minimise the time between students performing an activity and giving feedback
- try to balance negative comments with positive ones
- be constructive by indicating to students how they can improve
- fit feedback on assessed activity to the assessment criteria.

Remember that feedback can be given orally or in writing.

ACTIVITY 1.5

Feedback is an important aspect of learning and teaching. This activity asks you to reflect upon giving feedback.

You have observed that a student has not explained a procedure to an individual before starting to carry out the procedure.

What feedback might you give to the student?

How would you know if your feedback was effective?

What key principles would you use to inform the level and nature of feedback given to students? (This may be useful to include in your portfolio.)

Motivation

Motivation is a pivotal concept in the teacher role. It is closely related to arousal, attention, anxiety, and feedback/reinforcement. For example, a person needs to be motivated enough to pay attention while learning, and anxiety can decrease motivation to learn. Receiving a reward or feedback for an action usually increases the likelihood that the action will be repeated. Behavioural theories tended to focus on extrinsic motivation such as rewards, while cognitive theories deal with intrinsic motivation, i.e. goals.

Malone (1981) presented a theoretical framework for intrinsic motivation in the context of designing computer games for instruction. Malone argues that intrinsic motivation is created by three qualities: challenge, fantasy and curiosity. Challenge depends upon activities that involve uncertain outcomes due to variable levels, hidden information or randomness. Fantasy should depend upon skills required for the instruction. Curiosity can be aroused when learners believe their knowledge structures are incomplete, inconsistent or unparsimonious. According to Malone, intrinsically motivating activities provide learners with a broad range of challenge, concrete feedback and clear-cut criteria for performance.

Reigeluth and Carr-Chellman (2009) present an instructional design model for motivation that is based upon a number of other theories. Their model suggests a design strategy that encompasses four components of motivation: arousing interest, creating relevance, developing an expectancy of success and producing satisfaction through intrinsic/extrinsic rewards.

Authority

Teachers who have a formal authority approach to their role tend to focus on content. This style is generally teacher-centred, where the teacher feels responsible for providing and controlling the flow of the content and the student is expected to receive the content.

Teachers with this approach are not as concerned with building relationships with their students nor is it as important that their students form relationships with other students. This type of teacher doesn't usually require much student participation and may not promote student learning.

A number of teaching roles that the work-based facilitator could consider using have been identified and are described below.

Demonstrator or personal role

Teachers who have a demonstrator or personal model role tend to run teacher-centred classes with an emphasis on demonstration and modelling. This type of teacher acts as a role model by demonstrating skills and processes and then as a coach/guide who helps students develop and apply these skills and knowledge.

Teachers using this role tend to be interested in encouraging student participation and adapting their presentation to include various learning styles. Students are expected to take some responsibility for learning what they need to know and for asking for help when they don't understand something.

Facilitator

Teachers who have a facilitator role tend to focus on activities. This teaching style emphasises student-centred learning and there is much more responsibility placed on the students to take the initiative for meeting the demands of various learning tasks.

This approach works best for students who are comfortable with independent learning and who can actively participate and collaborate with other students.

Teachers typically design group activities that necessitate active learning, student-to-student collaboration and problem-solving. This role often involves designing learning situations and activities that require student processing and application of materials in creative and original ways.

Delegator

Teachers who have a delegator role tend to place much control and responsibility for learning on individuals or groups of students.

Those assuming this role will often give students a choice in designing and implementing their own complex learning projects and will act in a consultative role.

Students are often asked to work independently or in groups and must be able to maintain motivation and focus for complex projects. Students working in this type of setting learn more than just course specific topics as they also must be able to work effectively in group situations and manage various interpersonal roles.

ACTIVITY 1.6

This activity identifies the student as an active learner and challenges you to look at your role in this active process.

Students are required to meet course learning outcomes whilst in the workplace. Your role is to facilitate this active process. How would you involve students in identifying learning opportunities as part of this learning process?

What are the strengths of this partnership and why?

What action would you take to ensure that the students' learning outcomes are met? (This may be useful to include in your portfolio.)

Being an effective teacher

Often the work-based facilitator needs to reflect upon her/his role to analyse how effective s/he has been as a teacher. Greenaway (2012) believes that this can be a two-, three- or four-stage process. A two-stage learning cycle involves doing, i.e. experience, and then reviewing, i.e. reflecting.

The three-stage learning cycle involves experience and review, followed by identification of learning that will be applied to the next student activity. However, the four-stage model appears to be the basis of most experiential learning perspectives on the teacher role. This consists of:

- experience
- reflective observation
- conceptualisation
- experimentation.

Underpinning all these roles is the need to be a good teacher. This entails passion, not only motivating students to learn, but also teaching them how to learn, and doing so in a manner that is relevant, meaningful and memorable. Good teaching is also about substance and treating students as consumers of knowledge, striving to bridge the gap between theory and practice in the workplace. A good teacher listens, questions, responds and remembers that each student is different. It's about eliciting responses and developing the oral communication skills of the quiet students. It's about pushing students to excel; at the same time, it's about being human, respecting others and being professional at all times.

Another important feature of the role is not always having a fixed agenda and being rigid, but being flexible, fluid and experimenting and having the confidence to react and adjust to changing circumstances. Learning situations in the workplace can often change, which means that good teachers are confident enough to deviate from the session plan when the situation dictates or if there is more and better learning elsewhere.

It is also useful to remember that the role benefits from the use of humour, for example being self-deprecating and not taking oneself too seriously. It's often about making innocuous jokes, mostly at your own expense, so that the ice breaks and students learn in a more relaxed atmosphere.

The role also needs a nurturing component that seeks to develop students' minds and talents whilst on a work-based placement. Facilitators need to devote time, often invisible, to every student, such as preparing learning materials and organising a meeting with a colleague.

The most effective work-based facilitators can often demonstrate certain features in their role. Whilst generalising is difficult, there are some principles that may enhance work-based teaching and so promote student learning during placements.

- Respond to students' needs.

Teaching is most effective when it occurs in quick response to students' needs. So, even when occupied with something else, you should make every effort to teach the student(s) when asked. The student is ready to learn. Satisfy that immediate need for information now, and augment your teaching with more information later.

- Involve students in planning.

Just presenting information to students does not ensure learning. For learning to occur, you will need to get students involved in identifying their learning needs and outcomes. Help them develop attainable objectives. Give students the chance to test their ideas, to take risks and to be creative, as these will promote learning.

- Begin with what students know.

Learning is more rapid when it builds on what students already know. Teaching that begins by comparing the old, known information or process and the new, unknown one allows students to grasp new information more quickly.

- Move from simple to complex.

Students find learning more rewarding if they have the opportunity to master simple concepts first and then apply these concepts to more complex ones. Note, what one student finds simple, another may find complex. A careful assessment takes these differences into account and helps you plan the starting point for a session.

- Make material meaningful.

Another way to facilitate learning is to relate material to the students' life experiences. The more meaningful material is to students, the quicker and easier it will be learned.

- Allow immediate application of knowledge.

Giving the student the opportunity to apply new knowledge and skills reinforces learning and builds confidence. Immediate application of knowledge translates learning to the real world and provides an opportunity for problem-solving, feedback, and emotional support.

- Plan periodic rests.

Whilst you may want students to push ahead until they have learned everything on the teaching plan, periodic plateaus are a naturally occurring phenomenon. Students may feel overwhelmed and appear unreceptive to your teaching if student activity is particularly complex or lengthy. Try to recognise these signs of mental fatigue and let students relax. You can use these periods to review your lesson plan and make necessary adjustments.

- Tell students how they are progressing.

Learning is made easier when students are aware of their progress. Positive feedback can motivate them to greater effort because it makes session goals attainable. Also, ask students how they feel they are doing. They probably want to take part in assessing their own progress toward learning outcomes, and their input can guide your feedback.

The following website contains a range of activities that can be used for providing feedback: http://reviewing.co.uk/learning-cycle/feedback-methods.htm.

- Reward learning with praise.

Praising achievement of learning outcomes improves the chances that students will retain the material. Praising your students' successes associates the desired learning outcome with a sense of growing and accepted competence. Reassuring students that they have learnt desired material or technique helps students retain and refine acquired knowledge/skill.

ACTIVITY 1.7

This activity is designed to help you identify students' learning and what you feel is the best way to deliver that learning.

What are the tasks that you teach students whilst learning in your workplace?

What are the skills you want students to develop?

What attitudes do you try to get students to develop?

Reflect on how you deliver the attitude, skills and knowledge to students in the context of your workplace. Create a teaching and learning plan that on reflection will enable you to improve on the process of student learning in the workplace. (This may be useful to include in your portfolio.)

Teaching methods and techniques

A fundamental principle of work-based teaching is to create an environment that is encouraging and supportive of students engaging in the appropriate and necessary mental activity. This can be achieved by providing specifications of what the students must become able to do: set up or suggest activities that students can use to achieve intended learning outcomes. There are a number of teaching methodologies that can help work-based teachers achieve this goal.

Learning contracts

Atherton (2010) provides detailed information about the use of learning contracts, which are agreements between a teacher or teaching team and a learner or occasionally a group of learners. They normally concern issues of assessment and provide a useful mechanism for reassuring both parties about whether a planned piece of work will meet the requirements of a placement. It is based on the principle of the learners being active partners in the teaching-learning system, rather than passive recipients of whatever it is that the teacher thinks is good for them. It is about student ownership of the process.

The use of learning contracts does not automatically bring about this ownership and involvement. There is a risk that the contractual bargain is often one-sided, with all the obligations being on the side of the student, and none on the part of the teacher. The teacher does not even undertake unequivocally to award a pass mark to the resultant work: s/he will do so only if in her judgement it meets the required criteria. For example, the teacher undertakes that if the student produces such work as the teacher specifies, to a standard which the teacher will determine (whether or not that standard is based on fixed criteria or personal whim, and regardless of whether the standard is known to the student), the teacher will award a mark to that work. The student indicates acceptance of this 'agreement' by producing the work.

To avoid this, learning contracts should seek to make explicit this implicit deal, which should at least expose any one-sidedness and ideally provide a basis for addressing it. The following represents a useful example.

ACTIVITY 1.8

This activity reviews the use of learning contracts as a tool to facilitate learning and assessment.

Do you have a learning contract for students when they start learning in your workplace placement?

If yes, what are the benefits of having a learning contract?

What improvements can you make to the learning contracts you use? (This may be useful to include in your portfolio.)

If you have not created one, then create a learning contract for students starting placement with you. (This may be useful to include in your portfolio.)

Problem-based learning

A good starting definition of problem-based learning (PBL) is that the learning starts from a problem, a question or scenario, within which a number of themes or dimensions of learning are present. In most versions of PBL students would work together in groups, with the help of a facilitator, using 'problems' or scenarios as a basis for study. They share their existing knowledge and understanding relevant to the scenario, agree what they need to learn and how they will do this (drawing on a range of resources) and reconvene to discuss progress, evaluate their work and decide next steps. The scenarios often run over several weeks, during which the group may meet 4–6 times (Burgess 2006).

The principal aims of PBL are, according to Busfield and Peijs (2012):

- to integrate knowledge and skills from a range of multidisciplinary modules
- to acquire knowledge through self-study
- to teach students how to work in groups and manage group projects
- to improve and develop transferable skills of students
- to develop problem-solving skills of students
- to encourage self-motivation, curiosity and thinking
- and finally, to make learning fun!

Students are recommended by Busfield and Peijs (2012) to follow a stepped plan approach in order to ensure that a systematic method of working is used for all the case studies. Thus, group meetings should be structured to conform to the following 7-Step Project Plan of PBL:

- Step 1: Explain unknown wording, statements and concepts.
- Step 2: Define the problem(s).
- Step 3: Brainstorm – analyse/try to explain the problem(s).
- Step 4: Make a systematic inventory of explanations.
- Step 5: Formulate self-study assignments.
- Step 6: Perform self-study assignments.
- Step 7: Report and evaluate on self-study. After each group meeting, the group formulates the next stage of the self-study assignments.

Enquiry-based learning

Another method is enquiry-based learning, which refers to forms of learning driven by a process of enquiry (Price 2003). This usually involves a deep engagement with a complex problem.

Enquiry-based learning does not simply involve students in creating a finished product such as a project report or dissertation. In such cases it is still possible for students to bypass any significant engagement with a process of enquiry. Instead, enquiry-based learning incorporates structures and forms of support to help students carry out enquiries.

There is a clear overlap with problem-based learning, in which the solution of a problem shapes the whole learning experience of the students, but enquiry-based learning as defined here covers a broader spectrum of approaches:

1 project-based activities
2 problem-based learning
3 product design projects in engineering
4 case-study projects in Business Studies drawn from real life, with students playing the role of consultants
5 creative projects in the arts, such as a film-production project in Media studies
6 field-mapping excursions in Geography and Geology
7 programme-long design projects in Architecture
8 development of a mathematical model of some aspect of the real world.

Group work

Students who work in cooperative groups often do better than those who work alone, or competitively. Working in a group can provide opportunities which, as an individual learner, are not so readily available:

* Another member of the group may have knowledge or experiencethat may help you.
* A sense of responsibility to fellow students can provide good motivation and encouragement – for example, you may be more likely to do the preparation work if you know that your other group members are depending on you for one aspect of the group task.
* More complex problems can be solved by breaking them down into separate tasks for group members – for example, a reading list could be shared out and group members make their notes available to others.
* Discussing a subject with others can often help your understanding.

A number of skills are developed whilst working as part of a team, such as:

* interpersonal skills, e.g. assertiveness, debating ability
* oral communication skills
* self-appraisal, i.e. thinking about your own performance/contribution to the group task

as well as specific skills related to the group task, such as:

* critical reading
* time management
* negotiation
* decision-making.

Group size, and mix, will probably change depending on the nature of the task. Whatever the situation, it is important to consider the group dynamics. In order to work effectively together, group members need to get to know one another, to appreciate each others strengths (and weaknesses!) and to decide how they can best work as a group.

Lindsay (2005) points out that a facilitator needs to be aware of group dynamics and a group's development. He also suggests that optimum group size for placement students is three or four.

So far we have covered a range of teaching methodologies. A feature of many of these approaches is the use of certain teaching methods. Some of these are particularly appropriate for work-based learning. Table 1.2 presents the strengths and limitations of various teaching methods and what teachers need to do when using them.

Table 1.2 Analysis of teaching methods

Method	Strengths	Limitations	Preparation
Lecture	• presents factual material in direct, logical manner • contains experience which inspires • stimulates thinking to open discussion • useful for large groups	• experts are not always good teachers • student normally passive • learning is difficult to gauge • communication is predominantly one-way	• needs clear introduction and summary • needs time and content limit to be effective • should include examples, anecdotes
Lecture with discussion	• involves students, at least after the lecture • students can question, clarify and challenge	• time may limit discussion period • quality is limited to quality of questions and discussion	• requires questions to be prepared prior to discussion
Brainstorm/ thought shower	• listening exercise that allows creative thinking for new ideas • encourages full participation because all ideas equally recorded • draws on students' knowledge and experience • spirit of congeniality is created • one idea can spark off other ideas	• can be unfocused • needs to be limited to 5–7 minutes • people may have difficulty getting away from known reality • if not facilitated well, criticism and evaluation may occur	• teacher selects issue • must have some ideas if student needs to be stimulated
Video	• entertaining way of teaching content and raising issues • keeps students' attention • looks professional • stimulates discussion	• can raise too many issues to have a focused discussion • discussion may not have full participation • only as effective as following discussion	• need to set up equipment • effective only if facilitator prepares questions to discuss after the show
Small group discussion	• allows participation of everyone • people often more comfortable in small groups • can reach group consensus	• needs careful thought as to purpose of group • groups may get side-tracked	• need to prepare specific tasks or questions for group to answer
Worksheet/ directed study	• allows students to think for themselves without being influenced by others • individual thoughts can then be shared in large group	• can be used only for short period of time	• teacher has to prepare handouts
Work with colleague	• personalises topic • breaks down student stereotypes	• may not be a good teacher	• contact colleague and coordinate • introduce colleague appropriately
Demonstration	• rapidly transmits topic • useful for teaching skills • useful in variety of work-based settings • follow up with student practice	• needs detailed preparation • requires appropriate resources • demonstrator needs to be competent at skill • inadequate time/resources for student practice	• prepare setting • resource(s) functioning

> **ACTIVITY 1.9**
>
> Designing a teaching plan for a student is central to good teaching practice. This activity requires you to plan teaching for your student/learner.
>
> Select a topic that you need to teach. Break it down into stages and put it into a time frame for a student learning in your workplace. (This may be useful to include in your portfolio.)

Skills in teaching

The more organised a work-based teacher is, the more effective their teaching, and thus learning, will be. Many work-based teachers undertake formal teaching sessions that need to be planned. There are different approaches to planning teaching situations, though certain common principles exist.

Three stages of planning such sessions are:

1 Pre-session preparation
  - learning outcome(s) for the session
  - session content
  - academic level
  - prior student knowledge/experience
  - available resources.
2 Session plan
  - session outcome
  - teaching method(s)
  - student activity, e.g. discussion, practice
  - content
  - materials required
  - evaluation of session.
3 Post-session
  - analyse evaluation
  - changes to the session
  - implications for other sessions.

Work-based facilitators who develop highly structured and detailed plans rarely rigidly adhere to them. Such rigidity would probable hinder, rather than help, the learning process. The elements of your lesson plan should be thought of as guiding principles to be applied as aids, but not blueprints. Preparation must allow for flexibility

However, the work-based teacher needs an array of skills to ensure effective teaching in both formal and informal teaching situations. Some of the main skills are examined below.

Link student activity to learning style

A previous section of this unit considered different learning styles. An important skill is to be able to utilise a range of approaches to teaching, which has been based upon a student's learning style. For example, The Effective Teaching and Learning Network (2006) provide guidance on activity in relation to four learning styles.

The visual/verbal learning style

These students learn best when information is presented visually and in a written language format. In a formal setting, teachers should list the essential points of the session and provide an outline to follow during the session. Such students benefit from information obtained from articles, textbooks and notes. They tend to like studying alone in a quiet room.

The tactile/kinesthetic learning style

These students learn best when physically engaged in a 'hands-on' activity. In formal settings, teachers should allow students to manipulate materials to learn new information. Students with this learning style learn best when physically active in the learning environment. They benefit from instructors who provide demonstrations and 'hands-on' student learning experiences and allow students to participate in real work situations.

The auditory/verbal learning style

These students learn best when information is presented auditorily in an oral language format. In formal settings, they benefit from listening to the teacher and participating in group discussions. Such students also benefit from obtaining information from audio tape. When trying to remember something, they can often 'hear' the way someone told them the information, or the way they previously repeated it out loud. They learn best when interacting with others in a listening/speaking exchange.

Facilitation

Facilitation is often an important part of learning activities. In particular, facilitation is important in circumstances where people of diverse backgrounds, interests and capabilities work together (Information and Design 2012). An important aspect of the role of the work-based facilitator is to facilitate student learning. A facilitator is an individual whose job is to help to manage a process of information exchange. Good facilitation is hard work and it is difficult. There are many styles of facilitation and no single 'right' way to carry out the role. We each develop our own unique style and make different kinds of contribution to the facilitation function (Ward-Green and Hill 2012). Some key competencies in facilitation, based on the recommendations of various authors (Information and Design 2012, Ward-Green and Hill 2012) include:

- managing the relationship effectively by preparing thoroughly
- distinguishing process from content
- encouraging participation and creativity
- helping members to express and deal with conflict
- asking rather than telling
- maintaining objectivity
- being willing to spend time in building relationships rather than always being task-oriented
- encouraging quiet people to make contributions by asking them for their opinions and comments
- being attentive to what is happening at all times.

Questioning

Work-based facilitators may find that they need to ask students various types of questions. Most people think that questioning is so straightforward and easy that anyone can do it right (Nicholl and Tracey 2007). Nothing could be farther from the truth. Here are a number of simple guidelines to asking questions that should improve most teachers' questioning skills:

- Be sure that the question is clear in your own mind. Think through what you want from the student before you ask the question.
- Frame (state) the question without calling on a specific student. When you call on a student before the question is asked, every other student is free to ignore the question.
- After framing the question, pause while everybody has a chance to think of an answer, then (and only then) call on a student to respond. That is called wait time, and it is amazing how few teachers use this important questioning skill. The average wait time, when the teacher

waits at all after a question, is less than a second. There should be at least two to four seconds after any question before any student is called on to answer it. You might even try counting to yourself to force you to wait an appropriate time.

- Ask only one question at a time. Multiple-part questions are confusing and are likely to result in student misunderstanding. Avoid asking a series of related questions or restating the same question over and over without getting (sometimes without allowing) an answer.
- Use recall questions first to be sure that the student has the knowledge.

Planning

- Sources of information
  - Who has done good work on the topic?
  - What is best source of information?
  - How will we obtain this information?
- Ordering activity
  - What tasks need to be completed?
  - How should we organise the order of these tasks?
  - How much time will each task take?
  - What resources do we need?
  - What will you do next?
- Objective-setting
  - What do you want to achieve?
  - Who should do what?
  - What is the main outcome?
  - What are the other outcomes?

Probing and clarifying

Nicholl and Tracey (2007) also offer guidance on the use of probing as a questioning technique, believing that effective use of probing is one of the most important questioning skills. If the student does not provide a complete answer, he or she may know a partial answer. In some cases, even though the question is perfectly clear to the teacher, it might need to be restated or broken down into smaller pieces. The teacher should not accept 'I don't know' as the final response.

Probing is the use of further questions to force the student to put together his or her partial knowledge into a more complete answer. Probing often involves the use of follow-on or leading questions to help the student answer the initial question or to provide a more complete answer.

Probing means going deeper; it means digging. It can sometimes be painful to both the student and the teacher. It requires patience on the part of the teacher. In any case, it means not answering your own questions until you have tried to make the students think through the answer. Even a simple recall question may lead to important new learning on the part of the students if probing is used effectively.

- Relevance
  - What information should be retained?
  - How reliable is the information?
  - How can main findings be summarised?
- Clarifying
  - What does the information mean?
  - What assumptions underpin the information?
  - Is the information valid?
  - What would happen if you ... ?
- Elaborating
  - What does it mean?
  - How can something be taken further?
  - What does this mean for the task?

- How did you do that?
- Creative probing
  - What does this really mean?
  - What is missing?
  - How can information be regrouped?
  - What might you do instead?
- Provocative probing
  - What is the point of this?
  - Can we trust the information?
  - What if we do nothing?

The Active Listening (2006) website offers advice on other questioning techniques, such as those described below.

Paraphrasing

Paraphrasing involves restating a message, but usually with fewer words. Where possible try and get more to the point. It allows a facilitator to test understanding of what they heard. It communicates that the facilitator is trying to understand what is being said. If you're successful, paraphrasing indicates that you are following the student's verbal explorations and that you're beginning to understand the basic message.

When listening, consider asking yourself:

- What is the speaker's basic thinking message?
- What is the person's basic feeling message?

Examples include:

S: I just don't understand, one minute she tells me to do this, and the next minute to do that.
X: She really confuses you.

S: I really think he is a very nice guy. He's so thoughtful, sensitive, and kind. He calls me a lot. He's fun to go out with.
X: You like him very much, then.

Perception-checking

This is a request for verification of your perceptions. Facilitators can use perception-checking to give and receive feedback as well as check out your assumptions. Possible questions are:

'Let me see if I've got it straight. You said that you love your children and that they are very important to you. At the same time you can't stand being with them. Is that what you are saying?'

Summarising

Summarising involves pulling together, organising, and integrating the major aspects of your dialogue. Pay attention to various themes and emotional overtones. Put key ideas and feelings into broad statements. Do not add new ideas. It gives facilitators a sense of movement and accomplishment in the exchange, establishes a basis for further discussion and pulls together major ideas, facts and feelings. One way of summarising might be:

'A number of good points have been made about rules for the classroom. Let's take a few minutes to go over them and write them on the board.'
'We're going all over the map this morning. If I understand you correctly...'
'The three major points of the report are...'

Evaluating

- Show me what you might do with the information.
- How did you do that?
- What will you do when you have finished?
- How well does it function?
- Have you achieved the outcome(s)?
- What went well?
- What would you do differently?
- What would you tell someone else performing a similar task?

ACTIVITY 1.10

This activity builds upon the previous activity to plan and deliver a teaching session. Reflect upon the effectiveness of the teaching session by doing the following:

Video the teaching session.

On watching the video of the session, what are your strengths?

What areas require further development?

What action could you take to develop these areas? (This may be useful to include in your portfolio.)

Dealing with difficult students

ACTIVITY 1.11

Dealing with difficulties in teaching and students' learning will be something that you will occasionally encounter. This exercise is designed so that you may consider some of the actions you may take and why.

Think about any actual or potential difficulties in teaching that you have experienced or think possible in your workplace.

What action might you have/have you taken and how effective might these actions be/have they been in dealing with difficult students?

How, on reflection, could you improve when working with students in relation to the difficulties? (This may be useful to include in your portfolio.)

One situation that can be problematic for a work-based facilitator occurs when a placement student demonstrates difficult behaviour(s). The list below contains descriptions of some of the more commonly encountered examples of student behaviour as well as some possible strategies for dealing with difficult behaviour.

Rambling: wandering around and off the subject; using far-fetched examples or analogies

- Refocus attention by restating a relevant point.
- Direct questions to the group back onto the subject.
- Ask how the topic relates to the current topic being discussed.
- Say: 'Would you summarise your main point, please?' or 'Are you asking...?'

Shyness or silence: lack of participation

- Give strong positive reinforcement for any contribution.
- Involve by directly asking him/her a question.
- Make eye contact.
- Appoint to be small group leader if using group work.
- Don't over-pressurise.

Talkative: knowing everything, manipulation, chronic whining

- Acknowledge comments made.
- Give limited time to express viewpoint or feelings, and then move on.
- Make eye contact with another participant and move toward that person.
- Say: 'That's an interesting point. Now let's see what other people think', if appropriate, for example in a group situation.

Sharpshooting: trying to shoot you down or trip you up

- Admit that you do not know the answer and redirect the question back to the student.
- Acknowledge that this is a joint learning experience.
- Ignore the behaviour.

Arguing: disagreeing with everything you say; making personal attacks

- Recognise participant's feelings and move on.
- Acknowledge positive points.
- Say: 'I appreciate your comments', or 'It looks like we disagree.'
- Speak to student privately.

Overt hostility/resistance: angry, belligerent, combative behaviour

- Hostility can be a mask for fear. Reframe hostility as fear to depersonalise it.
- Respond to fear, not hostility.
- Remain calm and polite.
- Don't disagree, but build on or around what has been said.
- Move closer to the hostile person, maintain eye contact.
- Always allow student a way to gracefully retreat from the confrontation.
- Say: 'You seem really angry. Does anyone else feel this way?' Solicit peer pressure if relevant.
- Do not accept the premise or underlying assumption if it is false or prejudicial.
- Allow individual to solve the problem being addressed. He or she may not be able to offer solutions and will sometimes undermine his or her own position.
- Ignore the behaviour.

Griping: legitimate complaining

- Point out that we can't change policy here.
- Validate student's point.
- Indicate time pressure.
- Talk to student privately.

Designing a placement learning programme

There are a number of considerations when designing a placement learning programme. Whilst the nature of this programme may be predetermined by the students' college/university, it may be developed in collaboration with work-based placement providers or may even be left up to individual work-based facilitators to develop. The following features of a placement learning programme are fundamental to ensuring that the students undertake an effective programme.

Aims

The programme needs to have clear aims as this will guide both work-based facilitator and student. The aims should be specified in terms of the general aim of the teaching in relation to the placement. They should be broad or general statements of educational intent and indicate the overall purpose or desired goal of a placement. Remember that this information will be released to students and so it should be written in 'student-friendly' language.

Examples

'This placement aims to develop confidence in handling numerical information by consideration of a range of basic techniques for acquisition, handling, analysis and interpretation of data.'

'To facilitate in the learner the ability, which can be utilised in practice, to interpret and discuss the applicability of life science theories to assessing and planning neonatal special and intensive nursing care.'

'To demonstrate and provide pointers for the resolution of conflict between fire safety and other design considerations such as access for disabled people, historic conservation of buildings, etc.'

'To provide students with an insight and understanding of the methods used in contemporary engineering.'

Most placements will also state learning outcomes, which consist of statements about what the student is expected to know and/or be able to do at the end of the placement. It is important that these are expressed in a way that reflects the appropriate level for the course being studied when the placement takes place. Bloom's taxonomy (Bloom 2001) is a useful guide.

Most universities describe aims on a scale going from Level 4 to Level 8. Level 4 outcomes are normally associated with Certificate level or first year of an undergraduate programme. Level 5 outcomes are normally associated with Diploma level or second year of an undergraduate programme. Level 6 outcomes are normally associated with Degree level or final year of an undergraduate programme.

Level 7 outcomes are normally associated with taught Postgraduate programmes, whilst Level 8 outcomes are associated with Doctoral programmes.

Level 4 outcomes might include:

Develop a rigorous approach to the acquisition of a broad knowledge base; employ a range of specialised skills; evaluate information using it to plan and develop investigative strategies and to determine solutions to a variety of unpredictable problems; and operate in a range of varied and specific contexts, taking responsibility for the nature and quality of outputs.

Bloom's Taxonomy Level 4

- Knowledge: define, repeat, record, list, recall, relate, state.
- Comprehension: translate, discuss, describe, recognise, explain, identify, locate, report, review.
- Application: apply, employ use, practice, illustrate, operate, schedule.

Level 5 outcomes might include:

Generate ideas through the analysis of concepts at an abstract level, with a command of specialised skills and the formulation of responses to well-defined and abstract problems; analyse and evaluate information; exercise significant judgement across a broad range of functions; and accept responsibility for determining and achieving personal and/or group outcomes.

Bloom's Taxonomy Level 5
All the previously mentioned Level 4 outcomes, plus:

- Analysis: distinguish, analyse, differentiate, appraise, calculate, experiment, test, compare, contrast, criticise, debate, question, relate, solve, categorise.

Level 6 outcomes might include:
Critically review, consolidate and extend a systematic and coherent body of knowledge, utilising specialised skills across an area of study; critically evaluate new concepts and evidence from a range of sources; transfer and apply diagnostic and creative skills and exercise significant judgement in a range of situations and accept accountability for determining and achieving personal and/or group outcomes.

Bloom's Taxonomy Level 6
All the previously mentioned Level 4 and 5 outcomes, plus:

- Synthesis: compose, plan, propose, design, formulate, arrange, assemble, construct, create, organise, manage.
- Evaluation: judge, appraise, evaluate, rate, compare, revise, assess, predict.

Level 7 outcomes might include:
Display mastery of a complex and specialised area of knowledge and skill, employing advanced skills to conduct research or advanced technical or professional activity for related decision-making including use of supervision.

Outcomes include all previous levels, though now with emphasis on analysis, synthesis and evaluation.

Syllabus

This will consist of an overview of the material that students would study on the programme. This will relate to the topic as well as the stage that a student is at during a course.

Teaching methods

This should explain how students will learn and how they are supported to achieve the learning outcomes of the placement programme. Work-based facilitators need to consider how their choice of teaching method(s) will enable students to meet the placement's learning outcomes. This involves developing a clear understanding of the relationship between teaching method and each learning outcome.

Kearsley (2012) believes that teaching needs to be sequential. However, this can be done in several ways. For example:

- simple to complex sequence
- determined by student knowledge base
- allow student to choose
- focus on learning outcomes
- adapt to students' experience and interests.

Assessment

The placement may have a formal assessment strategy, normally determined by, or in collaboration with, the students' college/university. However, whilst many courses do not have a formal assessment strategy for students during a placement; it can often be useful to think about how students can be made aware of their progress during the placement. This can involve feedback on their achievement of the learning outcomes for the placement.

It is worth noting that students undertaking formal assessments will tailor their activity to attempt to maximise their performance on the assessment. Therefore, it is worth ensuring that student learning activity is aligned to the assessment strategy, which should be designed so that it judges student performance for all of the placement's learning outcomes.

Evaluation

Finally, an important part of any placement learning programme is that it is evaluated. The two main questions that an evaluation will help answer are:

1 How well am I teaching?
2 How can I improve students' placement experience?

There are a number of sources of information that can help inform the placement evaluation, including:

- students
- peers
- yourself
- external observer.

An open approach, obtaining written and/or verbal evaluation data from students, is often most useful as it provides qualitative feedback that can inform development of the programme. Such an approach might include:

- nature of student learning during the placement
- usefulness of any supporting materials/visits
- enjoyable aspects of the placement
- difficulties encountered by the student
- ways of developing/improving the placement.

ACTIVITY 1.12

It is important that you receive feedback about your effectiveness as a teacher and facilitator. This activity assists you to think about the best way(s) to do this.

Design a method for gathering feedback from students, peers, yourself and an external observer.

Gather evidence from these sources. (This may be useful to include in your portfolio.)

Reflect on the feedback that you have gathered from a period of time in which you facilitated students.

Design an action plan that incorporates how you will address the feedback you have been given. (This may be useful to include in your portfolio.)

Conclusion

This section has considered various aspects of work-based teaching, including learning theory, learning styles, approaches to being an effective teacher in the workplace and designing a work-based learning-teaching programme. The next section explores how work-based facilitators can support students on a placement and thus facilitate effective student learning.

References

Active Listening *Improve Your Ability to Listen and Lead.* www.ccl.org/leadership/pdf/community/alpresentation.pdf

Atherton, J. S. (2010) *Learning Contracts*. www.learningandteaching.info/teaching/learning_contracts.htm

Bandura, A. (1977) *Social Learning Theory*. General Learning Press.

Bandura, A. (1997) *Self-efficacy: The Exercise of Control*. Freeman.

Bandura, A. (1973) *Aggression: A Social Learning Analysis*. Prentice-Hall.

Bandura, A. (1969) *Principles of Behavior Modification*. Holt, Rinehart & Winston.

Biggs, J. (2011) *Teaching for Quality Learning at University*. Open University Press.

Bloom, B. S. (2001) *Taxonomy of Educational Objectives: The Classification of Educational Goals*. Longman.

Bruner, J. (1960) *The Process of Education*. Harvard University Press.

Bruner, J. (1966) *Toward a Theory of Instruction*. Harvard University Press.

Bruner, J. (1973) *Going Beyond the Information Given*. Norton.

Burgess, H. (2006) *What is PBL?* http://strathprints.strath.ac.uk/32297

Busfield, J. and Peijs, T. (2012) *Learning Materials in a Problem Based Course*. www.materials.ac.uk/guides/pbl.asp.

Combs, A. W. (1982) Affective Education or None At All. *Educational Leadership* 39(7): 494–7.

Daloz, L. (1986) *The Mentor's Guide*. Jossey-Bass.

Entwistle, N. (1988) *Styles of Learning and Teaching*. David Fulton.

Felder, R. (1993) Reaching the Second Tier: Learning and Teaching Styles in College Science Education. *Journal of College Science Teaching* 23(5): 286–90.

Felder, R. M. and Silverman, L. K. (1998) Learning and Teaching Styles in Engineering Education. *Engineering Education* 78(7): 674–81.

Felder, R. M. and Brent, R. (2005) Understanding Student Differences. *Journal of Engineering Education* 94(1): 57–72.

Greenaway R (2012) *Learning Cycles*. http://reviewing.co.uk/research/learning.cycles.htm

Hibernia College (2012) *Overview of Learning Styles*. www.learning-styles-online.com/overview.

Information and Design (2012) *Facilitation Techniques*. www.infodesign.com.au/usabilityresources/general/facilitationtechniques.

Kearsley, G. (2012) *Explorations in Learning and Instruction: The Theory into Practice Database*. http://tip.psychology.org/index.html.

Knowles, M. (1975) *Self-Directed Learning*. Follett.

Knowles, M. (1984) *The Adult Learner: A Neglected Species*, 3rd edn. Gulf Publishing.

Kolb, D. A. (1984) *Experiential Learning: Experience as the Source of Learning and Development*. Prentice-Hall.

Lindsay, T. (2005) Group Learning on Social Work Placements. *Groupwork: An Interdisciplinary Journal for Working with Groups* 15(1): 61–89.

Malone, T. (1981) Towards a Theory of Intrinsically Motivating Instruction. *Cognitive Science* 5(4): 333–69.

Messick, S. (1978) *Individuality in Learning*. Jossey-Bass.

Nicholl, H. M. and Tracey, C. A. B. (2007) Questioning: A Tool in the Nurse Educator's Kit. *Nurse Education in Practice* 7(5): 285–92.

Nulty, D. D. and Barrett, M. A. (1996) Transitions in Students' Learning Styles. *Studies in Higher Education* 21(3): 333–45.

Price, B. (2003) *Studying Nursing Using Problem-based and Enquiry-based Learning*. Palgrave Macmillan.

Ramsden, P. (2003) *Learning to Teach in Higher Education*. Routledge.

Riegeluth, C. M. and Carr-Chellman, A. (2009) *Instructional Design Theories and Models* Volume 3. Routledge.

Rogers, C. R. (1969) *Freedom to Learn*. Merrill.

Rogers, C. R. and Freiberg, H. J. (1994). *Freedom to Learn*, 3rd edn. Merrill/Macmillan.

Scandura, J. M. (2012) *Structural Learning Theory*. www.instructionaldesign.org/theories/structural-learning.html

Skinner, B. F. (1950) Are Theories of learning Necessary? *Psychological Review* 57(4):193–216.

Skinner, B. F. (1953). *Science and Human Behavior*. New Macmillan.

Skinner, B. F. (1957) *Verbal Learning*. Appleton-Century-Crofts.

Skinner, B. F. (1988) *Beyond Freedom and Dignity*. Harmondsworth.

The Effective Teaching and Learning Network www.etln.org.uk/master.pdf

Ward-Green, G. and Hill, R. (2012) *Facilitation*. www.wghill.com/facilitate.htm

Supporting learning in the workplace

Introduction

A key aspect of the work-based facilitator role is to support students through the placement. Facilitators need to know the skills required and the different learning environments in which learning opportunities are provided so that effective learning in the workplace occurs.

Aim of unit

This unit aims to prepare you for your role in supporting the learner in the workplace and to develop your understanding of the roles and responsibilities of a work-based facilitator.

Outcomes of the unit

At the end of this unit you will be able to:

1 appraise the roles and responsibilities of individuals associated with teaching and learning in the workplace
2 differentiate between different learning environments
3 demonstrate the skills required to effectively support learning in the workplace
4 Evaluate your role in providing support for learning.

Role and responsibilities

ACTIVITY 2.1

This activity will help you focus on your role of work-based facilitator and the skills and knowledge you need to be effective in this role.

Does your job description include the role of supporting learning and assessment in the work place?

If yes, how does it describe this role?

If no, how is your role recognised as part of your job?

How were you selected and trained for your role?

Reflect on whether the process was positive or negative.

Identify the knowledge and skills you feel you may need to be effective in this role.

Connecticut Learns (2012) states that a workplace facilitator serves as a coach, role model and advocate to the student, whilst the student learns and practises expected work behaviours (such as timely attendance, meeting deadlines and quality performance standards). The facilitator acts as an 'information broker', providing occupational and industry information to students to help them make appropriate career choices and be successful in the workplace. Helping students understand the unique 'culture' of an organisation is a key factor in successful workplace experiences. Workplace facilitators also help students understand the value of each task, how their work contributes to or influences the goals of the organisation, and how workplace requirements relate to what they are learning in the higher education institution, i.e. linking theory to practice.

A number of authors, including Burrill *et al.* (2010), Connecticut Learns (2012) and Sharp *et al.* (2010), have identified various features of the work-based facilitator role in supporting learning in the workplace:

- provide the student with an overview of the business, division functions and workplace rules, policies and procedures (including work-ethic issues, the organisational culture, unwritten rules and the social aspects of work)
- explain the organisation's goals to the student and discuss how each division contributes to the achievement of goals
- help the student understand his or her job responsibilities
- contribute to the design, development and objectives of the student's individual work-based learning plan
- guide the student in work-related decision-making, goal-setting, prioritising and scheduling
- assist with planning how learning outcomes might be achieved
- arrange for additional practical experience
- manage access to libraries or other learning resources available in the workplace
- coach in or demonstrate practical skills
- assist the student in identifying and developing specific occupational, technical skills and the core academic and employability skills
- help the student see connections between classroom learning and the workplace
- point out the differences between school and work environments, including acceptable behaviour and performance expectations
- help build the student's self-esteem and confidence by providing opportunities for success in the workplace and positively reinforcing accomplishments
- provide feedback necessary for the student to perform effectively, highlighting strengths and opportunities for growth and correcting inappropriate behaviour
- seek out the student's opinions and suggestions
- formally or informally evaluate the student's work performance
- coach the student to continuously improve work performance and encourage ongoing self-assessment
- help the student to realistically review their performance
- give the student a lift when morale is low
- make yourself available to listen and advise
- help the student to resolve conflicts, clarify issues and cope with stressful situations
- act as a liaison between workplace and higher education institution staff, mediating when necessary
- maintain communication with higher education institution staff concerning student's progress (may share this responsibility with workplace managers)
- model behaviours that lead to workplace success, including respectful communication and cooperation with colleagues
- evaluate self and student.

ACTIVITY 2.2

List four personal qualities that you feel you need to support a student learning in the work-place.

In practical terms, the features of the facilitator's role listed above can be put into the following four categories.

Manager

- liaison with university and service colleagues
- managing the learning environment
- planning student's programme
- carrying out student briefing
- dealing with conflict, difficulties
- managing student withdrawal from the placement.

Advisor

- identification of problems
- understanding that professional practice requires an educational relationship, not a thera-peutic one
- addressing student's problems where appropriate
- seeking additional help, where appropriate.

Educator

- identification of student's stage of development
- knowledge of learning styles
- awareness of learning theories, concepts of reasoning in the workplace
- negotiation of learning objectives or contract with student
- facilitation through reflection
- provision of on-going feedback and regular supervision sessions.

Assessor

- knowledge of assessment scheme and forms
- understanding of grading system, if applicable
- being able to judge and verify a student's level of competence
- dealing with a failing student.

Some of the attributes of an effective facilitator include:

- Enthusiasm – show genuine interest in the learner and his/her needs, aspirations and dreams.
- Motivation – encourage the learner to channel their energy into constructive change, new challenges and overcoming problems/difficulties in learning activity.
- Openness – share your experiences with the learner, being honest about yourself and the learner.
- Empathy – appreciate how a learner thinks, feels and behaves.
- Positivity – help learners to find solutions to learning difficulties.
- Listening – focus on what learner is saying so that your own thoughts don't crowd your interpretation of a situation.

ACTIVITY 2.3

Write a job description for your role as a facilitator of learning and assessment in the workplace including your key responsibilities and tasks.

You should consider how this role fits in relation to reporting structures, e.g. your workplace, the higher education institution.

How much time should you allocate on a weekly basis to each individual student and on what will you be spending the time, e.g. on-the-job training, supervision meetings, assessment?

You may want to include your current job description in your portfolio as well as an updated job description that includes your role as a facilitator of learning and assessment in the workplace.

A number of the features of the work-based facilitator's role will be dealt with in other units, for example facilitating reflection, giving feedback to failing students, assessment techniques and meeting the needs of students with a disability. This unit focuses on more general aspects of the role in supporting learning and assessment in the workplace.

The unit will now consider the responsibilities of the effective work-based facilitator who will often be responsible for identifying learning opportunities that may not be available in the primary location for the student placement.

ACTIVITY 2.4

What expectations do you think a student may have of you as their facilitator?

Before the student starts:

- Find out:
    - when the student is starting
    - what course they are on (diploma, degree)
    - what stage the student is at in their course
    - what type of prior work-based experience they might have.
- Make sure you are familiar with any of the course-related documentation, e.g. assessment form(s) and learning outcome booklet.
- Arrange your diary so that you can meet the student on their first day as students feel that this is really important.

Once the student has started:

- Negotiate how often you will meet to review progress.
- It is important to set time out from the day-to-day work activity to discuss with the student their progress, assessment arrangements and particular issues that the student or you might have.
- Identify what the content of these meetings will be.
- Draw up a structured programme for the student.
- Agree how often you will work with the student.

Students understand the value of good support and expect to:

- be challenged
- be coached

- receive support and encouragement
- develop a friendly relationship
- learn how the organisation works
- develop critical thinking
- learn from example
- learn from their mistakes
- obtain wise advice
- listen and be listened to
- develop self-awareness
- develop self-confidence
- develop their careers.

You may need to adapt your working style to meet the needs of a student coming to learn in your workplace whilst on placement. There may be many decisions to be made and activities to be planned before the first meeting with learners (Sisco 1991). One of the first is development of a statement that describes the workplace experience's purposes, the teaching methods, and how and why the experience will contribute to personal as well as professional development.

Sharp *et al.* (2010) provide some useful tips for the first meeting with the student, as listed below:

Practical aspects

- Identify when you can work together and identify alternative arrangements if you cannot work together.
- Check any higher education institution prerequisites/requirements for the placement.
- Swap contact details.
- Give an overview of the placement, e.g. organisation, functions, key personnel.
- Discuss any dress requirements/policies.
- Talk informally about what the student can/can't do on placement.
- Refer to the location of key policies and procedures including health and safety issues.
- Explain the routines of the placement/staff including hours/breaks.
- Introduce the student to key people.
- Discuss transport/parking, etc.
- Identify any available resources: libraries/computers/books, etc.
- Arrange for future meetings.

Start to build the relationship/initial meeting

- Tell the student about yourself as a person and a practitioner.
- Ask them about themselves as a person and as a student.
- Share previous experiences of 'supervising' and 'being a student'.
- Think about how you best like to facilitate learning – share 'top tips' for a successful relationship.
- Ask the student about their previous likes/dislikes about any previous placement relationships (what worked for them!).
- Find out about any anticipated blocks to their learning (see the unit on diversity for a discussion of what these might be).
- Discuss how you would like feedback on your performance and what opportunities there will be for that.
- How and when will you reflect on the learning experience?
- Discuss how to deal with problems and the associated responsibility/accountability.
- Start to think about action planning and goal- or objective-setting

Obtain background information about the student

- Ask if they have any particular support needs (see unit on diversity).
- Are they aware of support networks?
- What did the student do previously – prior placements/experiences?
- What previous feedback did they receive – how did they deal with it?
- What do they consider their specific strengths and areas for development (what have they previously enjoyed/avoided)?
- What do they want to experience/see/do/develop?
- What are their concerns regarding the placement – potential fears and anxieties?
- How do they usually achieve their goals – take responsibility?
- What do they have to achieve?
- What are their deadlines?

A useful device for organising the various learning materials a student may need to use is a workbook or study guide for the placement. An important advantage of creating a workbook or study guide is that it helps facilitate advanced planning and preparation for the various learning experiences a student may encounter during the placement. It also serves as an initial resource for both facilitator and student to update as needed. On a personal level, the workbook or study guide helps learners obtain a broad picture of the learning experience, and many appreciate having materials assembled in one convenient package.

Not only should the work-based facilitator prepare for the arrival of the student, but there should be a discussion about the nature of the student's workload during the placement as well as dealing effectively with their own workload. It is incumbent upon the work-based facilitator to ensure he/she has sufficient documentation from the higher education institution to enable the facilitator to act effectively as a work-based facilitator. The higher education institution will normally maintain close links with work-based facilitators, who need to accept responsibility for reporting any problems that might occur (Burrill *et al.* 2010).

It is good practice to record student attendance. The work-based facilitator then needs to take responsibility for alerting the relevant member of staff in the student's higher education institution if the student has a poor attendance record. The higher education institution can then investigate the reasons for the student's behaviour.

This section has considered the individual roles and responsibilities of the work-based facilitator in ensuring effective placement learning. The next section considers how the learning environment can also be an important determinant of workplace learning as well as the usefulness of learning contracts in enabling work-based facilitators to create an effective learning environment.

ACTIVITY 2.5

You have been asked to facilitate a student's learning for a four-week placement in your workplace.

Draw up a checklist of tasks and materials to be completed before a student starts placement with you.

Reflect on whether the checklist was effective once the placement has started.

What changes would you make to this checklist? (This could be useful in your portfolio.)

Learning environments

The Quality Assurance Agency (2010) code of practice for placement learning states that an effective placement learning opportunity is one in which the aims and intended learning outcomes are clearly defined and understood by all parties and where the responsibilities of the higher education institution, placement provider and student are made explicit. Whilst this statement identifies the basis for establishing an effective learning environment, it doesn't identify different types of learning environments that all have the potential to facilitate effective learning.

Middlesex University (2010) identifies different aspects of an effective learning environment, as described below.

Learner centred

- What does the learner bring to the learning setting? These may be beliefs, cultural background or knowledge of the academic content. This is what new information needs to be connected to.
- Learners use current knowledge to construct new knowledge and what they know and believe at the moment affects how they will interpret new information.
- Current knowledge can help or hamper learning.
- Teachers have a harder time in using the learner's background because they are not familiar with it. A teacher must make an effort to learn about their students' backgrounds if they are to effectively connect to their prior knowledge.

Knowledge centred

- Instruction that focuses on how to help students use their current knowledge and skills to think and solve problems.
- How do we help students learn and understand new knowledge versus learning a set of disconnected facts and skills?
- Too much information in the curriculum may result in developing disconnected facts or skills rather than connected knowledge.

Assessment centred

- Feedback is fundamental to learning – it may be the most powerful part of the learning experience.
- Students need opportunities for formative assessment that allow for revision and improvement of the quality of their thinking and understanding.
- If the learning goal is to enhance understanding and applicability of knowledge, it is not sufficient to provide assessments that focus primarily on memorizing facts and formulas.

Community centred

- The learning environment must promote a sense of community.
- Most activities outside school are based in community settings, homes, clubs, teams, etc.
- A community allows more opportunity for motivation, interaction, and feedback.

Whatever the learning environment, it is important for a work-based facilitator to set a positive tone during the first encounter with a student, since this is the time when students form personal attitudes about the workplace, the facilitator and the learning process (Sisco 1991). Three opening questions that could be used to facilitate dialogue with a student are:

Who are we?

Asking this question is a good way of helping a student to get to know the facilitator. The question and responses also help start the process of working together and creating a relaxed, informal environment.

Who am I as the facilitator?

In asking and answering this question, a facilitator can establish credibility and authenticity with the student by indicating his or her credibility in supervising the placement experience. A particularly productive way of answering is to describe one's educational and workplace background. This is also a good time to share personal beliefs about what constitutes good and bad workplace experience and how this placement will be a positive learning experience, even though there may be a good deal of personal challenge involved.

Why are we here?

This question is a good lead-in to describing the general focus of the workplace experience by touching on the overall experience, suggested objectives, and learning process.

ACTIVITY 2.6

Complete a SWOT analysis on the learning environment in your workplace, by using the form in Table 2.1, p. 68.

List the action you could take to improve the learning environment? (This could be useful in your portfolio.)

Clark (2010) believes that physical and psychological barriers to effective communication exist, which have the potential to have a detrimental effect upon the quality of the learning environment. For example:

- Culture, background, and bias. We allow our past experiences to change the meaning of the message. Our culture, background and bias can be good as they allow us to use our past experiences to understand something new, but it is when they change the meaning of the message that they interfere with the communication process.
- Noise. Equipment or environmental noise impede clear communication. The sender and the receiver must both be able to concentrate on the messages being sent to each other.
- Ourselves. Focusing on ourselves, rather than the other person, can lead to confusion and conflict. The 'Me Generation' is out when it comes to effective communication. Some of the factors that cause this are defensiveness (we feel someone is attacking us), superiority (we feel we know more than the other) and ego (we feel we are the centre of the activity).
- Perception. If we feel the person is talking too fast, not fluently, does not articulate clearly, etc., we may dismiss the person. Also, our preconceived attitudes affect our ability to listen. We listen uncritically to persons of high status and dismiss those of low status.
- Environment. Bright lights, a background activity, unusual sights or any other stimulus provide a potential distraction.
- Smothering. We take it for granted that the impulse to send useful information is automatic. Not true! Too often we believe that certain information has no value to others or they are already aware of the facts.
- Stress. People do not see things the same way when under stress. What we see and believe at a given moment is influenced by our psychological frames of references – our beliefs, values, knowledge, experiences and goals.

These barriers can be thought of as filters, that is, the message leaves the sender, goes through the above filters and is then heard by the receiver. These filters muffle the message. The way to overcome filters is through active listening and feedback, skills which we will consider at a later stage in this unit. One practical way of creating an appropriate learning environment is through the use of learning contracts.

ACTIVITY 2.7

Reflect on an initial meeting you had with a student concerning a learning contract. What were the positive and developmental aspects you highlighted?

What improvements could you make to initial meetings with students? (This could be useful in your portfolio.)

The use of a learning contract allows negotiation between the clinician and the student with regard to what is needed, what is wanted and what is possible (Congdon *et al.* 2010). They believe that, first, students may come to placements with little idea about what they could hope to learn during the placement, and their learning objectives may be unreasonable or unrealistic. The use of a learning contract allows clarification of what the student can expect to see/do/learn during a placement, and therefore lets them set more achievable goals.

Second, by discussing the learning contract, all involved in the learning process are aware of each others intentions for the learning experience, and therefore are working towards the same goals. This can reduce conflict and confusion during the placement. This enables facilitator and student to:

- look back over experiences and identifying the learning that has occurred
- look forward and plan how this learning will be applied in the future.

Formal review will occur in progress meetings as well as in the final meeting of the placement. Neither students nor facilitator should ignore other more informal opportunities. The main functions of progress and evaluation meetings are:

- to check progress in relation to learning outcomes
- to identify weaknesses that are hindering progress and to identify strengths
- to plan for the future and set or revise targets
- to agree the kind of support that you will provide.

Learning contracts should, according to Rae (2010):

- be simple and straightforward
- be clear and unambiguous
- contain items that can be implemented by the learner at work, with or without support
- identify any resources that might be available
- contain comments on the methods to be used; the resources required and the timings, e.g. start and finish times or dates, for all the action items (use 'SMART' – Specific, Measurable, Agreed, Realistic, Time-bound).

Suggested content of a learning contract should deal with the following points:

- What is the item of learning you intend to implement?
- By which targets will you measure progress?
- What barriers might impede your implementation?
- How will you avoid or negate these barriers?
- Time: when do you intend to start implementing the item?
- Time: by when do you intend to complete the implementation of the item?
- Resources: what resources (people, equipment, extra skills, etc.) will you need to complete the implementation of the item?
- Benefits: what benefits do you hope will result from your actions (including financial benefits, if possible to assess)?
- Any other comments?

A facilitator may want to use the following principles to enable effective use of a learning contract:

1 Discover what the student wants to learn

Students learn best when the subject under discussion has been identified by them as an area that they need help with. Occasionally students need help to identify what they want to learn within a certain topic. Exposure to particular problems, hypothetical situations, vignettes and role plays can all help students see what they want to learn.

2 Discover what the student needs to learn

Your assessment of the student's performance may identify areas for improvement that they have not recognised themselves. More commonly the student may feel inadequate in areas in which you feel they are thoroughly competent.

3 Negotiate the content, methods and priorities of the teaching session with the student

Even short informal teaching episodes need to be negotiated, including the content of the session, the time to be taken and the method to be used. If there are many areas identified as important for learning, priorities may also need to be negotiated.

4 Use appropriate methods and techniques in any teaching sessions

Different students learn best in different ways. Some prefer reading around topics, others learn best from experience with clients. The facilitator needs to take account of a student's preferred style of learning. In each learning situation the facilitator has responsibility to ensure that all the dimensions of a problem are explored. These may include, administrative issues, published evidence and audit as well as an awareness of the student's own values and attitudes to the problem. Students may not see enough of certain situations, so the teacher can draw out general principles from a specific situation which the student can apply to other situations.

5 Plans for further learning

At the end of a teaching session find out what has been learnt and what still needs to be learnt. This helps the student to see that progress in covering the planned content for the placement has been made. It also provides valuable feedback to the teacher and helps form plans for future learning activities.

6 Provide an environment throughout the placement that is complemented by examples of good practice that reinforces learning

This is particularly important when students are watching the facilitator go about his/her work. The facilitator not only needs to set a good example but to be able to describe its constituent parts to the student, indicating techniques that are helpful as well as those that are not.

7 Establish a relationship with the student that is practical and appropriate to the developmental stage of the student in the process of moving from being a dependent student to becoming an independent practitioner

8 Evaluate the teaching

Facilitators may have to alter their role in facilitating the implementation of the learning contract. It may need to be directive, i.e. telling the student what to do. Sharp *et al.* (2010) caution against using this approach, though recognise that it may be useful under certain circumstances during a work-based placement, e.g. when:

- aims and objectives are unclear and will be difficult to clarify
- there are very tight time constraints
- the culture/atmosphere is one of suspicion and insecurity
- the attitude towards information is one of limited access and concealment
- your facilitation skills are undeveloped.

A preferred approach is to be facilitative, namely to support students, remove obstacles to learning and create an environment for student-led progress. The skills of facilitation will be considered in the next section of this unit. A facilitative approach is particularly useful when:

- aims and objectives are crystal clear or are capable of clarification
- sufficient time is available or can be made available to meet the aims and objectives
- the culture/atmosphere is one of openness and trust
- the attitude towards information is one of accessibility and transparency
- you are confident in your facilitation skills.

The next section will consider the skills that a work-based facilitator should develop to ensure effective implementation of a learning contract.

Skills for supporting learning in the workplace

A key skill in being an effective work-based facilitator is, according to Burrill *et al.* (2010), being able to develop positive attitudes towards students as these will tend to have a beneficial effect on students' learning and attitude. In contrast, negative characteristics – being rigid, dominating, arrogant, uncaring, lacking in confidence, unsupportive, belittling – can have the opposite effect.

Furthermore, the work-based facilitator should be able to

- prepare/plan appropriate induction
- arrange a timetable for self/student/other members of the team where appropriate
- impart work-related skills
- share knowledge at the appropriate level and in an appropriate style
- assess – being non-threatening and open-minded
- observe
- communicate
- manage time in relation to workload and student
- reflect on own and student's performance
- support effectively through formal and informal supervision
- delegate appropriate work to the student
- identify stress and manage it effectively – your own and student's
- be able to give constructive support and criticism.

Ramaley (2009) identifies a number of key principles in supporting work-based learning, including:

1   Encourage active learning, i.e. students can talk about their learning, write about it, relate it to past experiences and apply it to the workplace.
2   Give prompt feedback, particularly by giving students frequent opportunities to perform and receive suggestions for improvement.
3   Emphasise the time to be spent on an activity; allocating realistic amounts of time builds effective learning for students and effective teaching during the placement.
4   Communicate high expectations, as expecting students to perform well becomes a self-fulfilling prophecy when facilitators hold high expectations of themselves and make extra efforts.

The effective work-based facilitator will, according to Connecticut Learns (2012), be:

- willing and able to commit the necessary time to a student
- interested in helping and teaching students
- able to communicate effectively with students
- able to see student supervision as an opportunity rather than a task
- sensitive to culturally diverse backgrounds
- capable of encouraging, supporting, motivating and leading others
- willing to share constructive criticism and feedback in a supportive, sensitive and patient manner.

Research by Gray and Smith (2000) identifies students' views on the features of effective student support:

- Support the student, rather than breathe down their neck.
- Encourage and allow involvement and participation in normal work activities rather than just observation.
- Show confidence in the student's abilities and trust them to do things unsupervised.
- Form a relaxed relationship with the student.
- Take time every day to let the student do or observe something and do not assume that they have already seen or performed it.
- Regardless of the student's stage in the programme, have an initial discussion, preferably on the first day, to determine what the student's present abilities are and their intended learning outcomes for the placement.
- Ascertain what the student requires as an individual to meet the required learning outcomes.
- Clarify ground rules on both sides and discuss the opportunities available to meet desired learning outcomes.
- Remember to tell the student if there is anything particularly interesting happening on the placement.
- Allow the student some independence by giving more guidance at the beginning of the placement and then standing back to let the student show initiative and self-motivation.
- If you are not at work, make arrangements with other members of staff to look out for them rather than have the student feel abandoned.
- Think carefully about organising your workload to allow opportunities for you and the student to work together.

ACTIVITY 2.8

What are the learning outcomes your student should meet as a result of being on a work placement with you?

Complete a learning contract that reflects these learning outcomes and your personal aims and objectives for the work placement. (This could be useful in your portfolio.)

There are certain specific skills that an effective work-based facilitator needs to ensure effective student learning during the placement. These are described below.

Presentation skills

Work-based facilitators often have to make presentations to students. The University of Newcastle (2009) has produced some information on effective presentations.

Preparation

Prepare the structure of the talk carefully and logically, just as you would for a written report. What are:

- the objectives of the talk?
- the main points you want to make?

Make a list of these two things as your starting point.

Write out the presentation in rough, just like a first draft of a written report. Review the draft. If there are things you cannot easily express, possibly because of doubt about your understanding, it is better to leave them unsaid.

Never read from a script. It is also unwise to have the talk written out in detail as a prompt sheet – the chances are that you will not locate the thing you want to say amongst all the other text. You should know most of what you want to say, therefore prepare *cue cards* which have key words and phrases (and possibly sketches) on them. Postcards are ideal for this. Don't forget to number the cards in case you drop them. Rehearse your presentation – to yourself at first and then in front of some colleagues.

Making the presentation

Greet the audience. Good presentations then follow this formula:

- tell the audience what you are going to tell them
- then tell them
- at the end, tell them what you have told them.

Stick to the plan for the presentation and don't be tempted to digress – you will eat up time and could end up in a dead-end with no escape! Leave time for discussion – 5 minutes is often sufficient to allow clarification of points. At the end of your presentation ask if there are any questions – avoid being terse when you do this as the student(s) may find it intimidating (i.e. it may come across as, 'Any questions? – If there are, it shows you were not paying attention.'). If questions are slow in coming, you can start things off by asking the students a question – have one prepared.

Delivery

Speak clearly. Don't shout or whisper – judge the acoustics of the room. Don't rush, or talk deliberately slowly. Be natural – although not conversational. Deliberately pause at key points – this has the effect of emphasising the importance of a particular point you are making. Avoid jokes – always disastrous unless you are a natural expert. To make the presentation interesting, change your delivery, but not too obviously, e.g. speed and pitch of voice.

Use your hands to emphasise points, but don't indulge in too much hand waving. People can, over time, develop irritating habits. Ask colleagues occasionally what they think of your style.

Look at the audience as much as possible, but don't fix on an individual – it can be intimidating. Pitch your presentation towards the back of the audience, especially in larger rooms. Keep an eye on the students' body language. Know when to stop and also when to cut out a piece of the presentation.

Visual aids

Visual aids significantly improve the interest of a presentation. However, they must be relevant to what you want to say. A careless design or use of a slide can simply get in the way of the presentation. What you use depends on the type of talk you are giving. Here are some possibilities:

- computer projection (PowerPoint, applications such as Excel, etc.)
- video and film

- real objects – either handled by the speaker or passed around
- flipchart or whiteboard.

Make sure that you know in advance how to operate the equipment and also when you want particular displays to appear.

ACTIVITY 2.9

Reflect on a presentation you have made to students. In light of the information given in this unit, can you revise this presentation to include specific improvements and include this presentation in your portfolio?

Identify any changes to the original presentation together with your reasons for making these changes. (This could be useful in your portfolio.)

Negotiation skills

The unit has previously discussed various aspects of supporting learning that may require negotiation between facilitator and student, e.g. learning contracts. Consequently, a work-based facilitator needs effective negotiation skills. Management Sciences for Health (2012) outlines a number of key steps that underpin use of effective negotiations:

- Analyse the interest of the parties as this is important to understand the perceptions, the style of negotiation and the interests and principles of the counterparts, as well as one's own.
- Plan the negotiation, and determine:
  - What are the expectations from the negotiation?
  - What are the terms of the negotiation?
  - What is non-negotiable and what can be modified?
  - What is the minimum that an agreement can be reached on?
  - What is the negotiation strategy?
  - What are the most important interests of the student?
  - How does one interact with or manage people?
- Select the appropriate negotiation technique from among the following:
  - Spiralling agreements. Begin by reaching a minimum agreement even though it is not related to the objectives, and build, bit by bit, on this first agreement.
  - Changing of position. Formulate the proposals in a different way, without changing the final result.
  - Gathering information. Ask for information from the student to clarify their position.
  - Making the cake bigger. Offer alternatives that may be agreeable to the student without changing the terms.
  - Commitments. Formalise agreements orally and in writing before ending the negotiation.
- Negotiate: be sensitive and quick to adapt to changing situations, but do not lose sight of the objective. Avoid confrontational positions and try to understand the student's interests. Some aspects that could interfere with the negotiation are:
  - personal positions and interests
  - psychological and emotional aspects of the persons involved (place, placement of chairs, body language, gestures, etc.)
  - difficulties in communication, e.g. differences in languages, different meanings of the same words.

Questioning skills

Most people think that questioning is so straightforward and easy that anyone can do it right. Nothing could be farther from the truth. Some simple guidelines to asking questions that should improve most work-based facilitators' questioning skills include:

- Be sure that the question is clear in your own mind. Think through what you want from the student before you ask the question.
- After framing the question, pause while the student has a chance to think of an answer, i.e. wait time. It is surprising how infrequently people use this important questioning skill. The average wait time after a question is less than a second. There should be at least two to four seconds after any question before a student answers it. To help you avoid answering, try counting slowly to four.
- Ask only one question at a time. Multiple-part questions confuse students and are likely to result in misunderstanding. Also avoid 'shotgun' questioning, i.e. asking a series of related questions or restating the same question over and over without getting (sometimes without allowing) an answer.
- Use recall questions first to assess whether the student has acquired the necessary knowledge before proceeding to comprehension and analysis questions. Follow these up with evaluation questions.

Wang and Ong (2003) believe that facilitators should ask the following types of questions.

Challenging questions

Avoid phrasing questions that are closed, which require straightforward factual answers, unless you simply want to check retention. Ask probing and evaluative questions that call for higher cognitive thinking such as analysis, synthesis and evaluation. Challenge students to explore the evidence for their existing knowledge, apply their existing knowledge to other situations and bring them to the limits of their knowledge base.

An example of a straightforward question is: What is the expression for kinetic energy?

An example of a more challenging question is: Why is there a factor of $\frac{1}{2}$ in the expression for kinetic energy?

Well-crafted, open-ended questions

To start an active discussion, ask open-ended questions that encourage the exploration of various possibilities. However, the questions should not be too unstructured as this may lead to ambiguity, and time is lost defining the question rather than addressing the issue at hand. Encourage students to figure out answers rather than remember them. At times questions are designed to help students see things from a broader perspective, but this may necessitate other questions along the way to help the students narrow their focus before arriving at the answer.

An example of an open-ended and structured question is: We have examined the causes of dental caries. What factors would increase a patient's risk to caries?

Ask uncluttered questions

Avoid cluttered questions that involve many sub-questions or are interspersed with background information. This type of question confuses students because they are not clear what is being asked of them.

An example of a cluttered question is: What are some of the reasons that Newton's laws are flawed? I mean ... what seems to be the main problem, according to Einstein? Can we then still use Newton's laws? A few of you earlier said that you do not think Newton's laws should be used for some situations. What are the problems there?

Brief examples of additional question types are:

- *Questions that seek clarification*
  e.g. Can you explain that?

- *Questions that probe reasons and evidence*
  e.g. Why do you think that?

- *Questions that explore alternative views*
  e.g. What would someone who disagreed with you say?

- *Questions that test implications*
  e.g. What follows from what you say?

- *Questions about questions/discussion*
  e.g. Do you have a question about that?
  e.g. Who can summarise so far?

Listening skills

Steps to attentive listening based on Cortright (2012) include:

- squarely face the person
- focus on what the person is saying
- minimise internal distracting thoughts
- maintain eye contact
- keep an open mind on what is being said.

The authors link good listening skills with development of empathy with the student and separate it into primary and advanced empathy. Primary empathy is the reflection of content and feelings. The purpose is:

- to show that you're understanding the student's experience
- to allow the student to evaluate his/her feelings after hearing them expressed by someone else.

Basic formula:

> You feel *(state feeling)* because *(state content)*

e.g.

Student: I just don't know how I am going to get all this maths homework done before tonight's game, especially since I don't get most of this stuff you taught us today.
Facilitator: You are feeling frustrated and stuck ... You are feeling frustrated and stuck with a task that you don't know how to do and you're worried that you won't figure it out in time. The main fear for you seems to be fear.

It's upsetting when someone doesn't let you tell your side of the story.

Advanced empathy is the reflection of content and feeling at a deeper level. The purpose is to try and get an understanding of what may be deeper feelings.

e.g.

> 'I get the sense that you are really angry about what was said, but I am wondering if you also feel a little hurt by it.'

> 'You said that you feel more confident about contacting employers, but I wonder if you also still feel a bit scared.'

Clark (2010) describes some of the traits of a good listener:

- Spends more time listening than talking.
- Does not finish the sentence of others.
- Does not answer questions with questions.
- Is aware of biases. We all have them…we need to control them.
- Never daydreams or becomes preoccupied with their own thoughts when others talk.
- Let's the other speaker talk. Does not dominate the conversation.
- Plans responses after the other person has finished speaking…NOT while they are speaking.
- Provides feedback, but does not interrupt incessantly.
- Analyses by looking at all the relevant factors and asking open-ended questions. Walks the person through their analysis (summarises).
- Keeps the conversation on what the speaker says…NOT on what interests them.
- Takes brief notes. This forces them to concentrate on what is being said.

Feedback skills

Another key aspect of the work-based facilitator's role is providing students with feedback. However, this may not always be done very well or is even avoided. There may be a number of reasons why facilitators avoid giving feedback. Kleffner and Hendrickson (2001) identify some:

- A facilitator may not feel comfortable providing feedback.
- Students are anxious about receiving feedback considered to be negative.
- Time is not always available for the facilitator to provide feedback.

The features of providing feedback, based on the work of Leading Insight (2012) include:

- Identify the problem clearly and specifically. Take the time to identify the problem clearly and then organise the issues that need to be addressed. Is this an isolated problem or can this be seen in many areas of their performance? How does this issue impact the success of the individual's performance? How does it impact the rest of the team/organisation?
- Select an appropriate time and place. Pick a time and place where you will not be interrupted, and where the environment is appropriate to the type of message you are delivering. Explain the value of feedback and that you want to give feedback to support the student's growth and learning.
- Setting the stage. Acknowledge that it is difficult to hear feedback. The most common error is for people to take the feedback personally, stop listening and become defensive. This does not allow for the person to easily change their behaviour. It is therefore useful to state that the feedback is about a specific behaviour, and not about them as a person.
- Describe the behaviour. Describe the behaviour that you see. Be specific and stick to the facts, e.g. 'You are consistently late to our team meetings.'
- Make your case. Detail the implications of how this issue affects others, one's-self, or the success of the company, e.g. 'When you are late to meetings, people do not see you as a committed student.'
- Hold your ground. If the student pushes back, you need to listen for new information, but hold your ground and continue to be specific until it is clear that the message is understood, e.g. 'I understand that you have been very busy recently, but your being late impacts the rest of the team who are also busy.' Often you may only need to go to this step for the person to get it and agree to change, in which case go to the final step in this list. If not, go further.
- Explore the issue fully. Before you can develop a plan for change you need to fully understand the total context in which the behaviour occurs, e.g. are you having difficulty managing your time effectively? At this stage the person receiving the feedback may offer a different interpretation of the behaviour or apologise and commit to changing their behaviour, e.g. 'My tardiness is due to a medical problem that requires time-sensitive injections.'

- Describe the positive consequences. To build a commitment to change, describe the positive consequences of the behaviour being addressed, e.g. 'If you arrive on time to our meetings, you will be accepted by the team and involved in the decision-making.' If there is now a commitment to change you can go to the final step.
- Describe the negative consequences. If the student is still pushing back, you will need to describe the negative consequences of the behaviour, e.g. 'If you continue to be late you will be placed on a performance plan and I will inform your higher education institution.' (This is an example of a consequence if no new information was discovered.) This model is useful if the person is prepared to listen and change. However, not everyone is open to receive feedback and willing to adapt their behaviour. If the student cannot use constructive feedback, you will need to decide whether you want to accept their behaviour or inform their higher education institution.
- Plan for change. The outcome of this process is a commitment and a plan to change. The plan should include agreement of the stated problem and a detailed action plan with milestones for progress reviews, e.g. 'As agreed, we will change your hours due to your medical condition and communicate to the team the need to change the timing of the team meeting to include you. Let us review if this is working in two weeks.'

ACTIVITY 2.10

Identify how you could be more assertive. You may find the following website helpful: http://www.mindtools.com/pages/article/Assertiveness.htm.

Facilitators also need to receive feedback from students. This requires the facilitator to:

- listen – if something helps you to listen do that, e.g. take notes, ask someone else to make notes on the feedback so that you can focus on the speaker
- ask questions to clarify – 'Could you give an example of that?', 'When did that happen?', 'Who else was there?
- acknowledge valid points
- open yourself. Do not get defensive (you may feel it, but don't act it). Stay focused on hearing what is being said.
- take time to think about what has been said; if a response is necessary, tell those offering the feedback that you will think about it and offer some response on a specific date.

Some possible feedback statements include:

'When you . . .'. Note the behaviour; describe it as specifically as possible.
'I felt . . .'. Tell how the behaviour affects you. This is just one or two words – frustrated, angry, pleased, etc.
'Because I . . .'. Share why you are affected that way.
'I would like . . .'. What you would like the person to consider doing.
'Because . . .'. Why you believe it will help.
'What do you think?' Invite and hear the response; explore options.

ACTIVITY 2.11

How do you ensure that you get feedback from students?

In what ways can you improve on the quality and quantity of feedback that you give students? (This could be useful to include in your portfolio.)

Teaching a skill

An important element of work-based teaching will be teaching students skills, which Sharp *et al.* (2010) break down into three fundamental components:

- Break down the skill
Although you can teach a skill as a whole, there are so many components that you and the student may agree that it is best learnt part by part, gradually integrating these into a single skill.

- Repeat and practise
Mastery is only acquired with repeated practice, so the facilitator must be clear what minimum standard of practice is acceptable to ensure safe performance.

- Resist the urge to intervene
Having placed the student in the role of novice practitioner, the facilitator must resist the urge to take over for reasons other than putting others, e.g. clients, colleagues, at risk. During the session students may feel exposed, vulnerable and anxious and will benefit from prompt and consistent feedback on their performance. This will help both you and the student to identify where they are with that particular skill acquisition.

Sharp *et al.* identify two models for teaching a skill. First, the Integrated Skills Teaching model, which has five stages:

Stage 1 – Exposure to an experience which involves a skill
The skill is demonstrated at normal speed as part of a scenario that represents a realistic situation or a real-life situation. This ensures that the students do not perceive the skill in isolation.

Stage 2 – Exploration and elaboration
There follows a teacher and student discussion, where the skill is explained and elaborated upon and links to theory are made more explicit. Within this stage students' previous experiences can be discussed in relation to any differences noted or personal experiences.

Stage 3 – Experimental stage
Students practise the skill in a systematic and critical way whilst observed by the facilitator who provides the students with feedback and reinforcement, which is vital for skill development.

Stage 4 – Evaluation
A short discussion takes place to evaluate and share experiences. The aim of this evaluation process is for students to ascertain their needs in relation to this skill and identify where they need to enter the cycle next time.

Stage 5 – Skill acquisition
The students then dip in and out of the cycle at varying points until skill acquisition has been achieved. Students will reach this point at varying times. Therefore, once skill acquisition has been achieved, the cycle has ended. However, continuing learning will occur in relation to the skills taught as they are used in the learning environment as practice evolves.

The second approach is the four-stage model:

Stage 1 consists of a demonstration of the skill at normal speed, normally with no explanation.

Stage 2 is repetition of the skill with full explanation, at the same time encouraging the student to ask questions. (A video approach can be used for the first two stages; this ensures consistency and is less resource-intensive, if used in a simulated environment.)

Stage 3 is where the facilitator performs the skill with the students providing the explanation for each step and being questioned on key issues to ascertain student understanding. This step can be repeated several times until the facilitator is happy that the student can link the theory to the skill.

Stage 4 is when the students practise the skill under close supervision, describing each step before it is taken. Students must be given constructive feedback and allowed time for reflection and practising the skills to ensure that learning takes place.

ACTIVITY 2.12

Take an example of a particular skill that you teach your students.

Describe the tasks involved in the skill, specifying what attitudes, skills and knowledge you would be covering and the standard when teaching this skill.

How will you teach this skill?

Why have you chosen this approach? (This could be useful to include in your portfolio.)

Facilitation skills

The term facilitator comes from the Latin 'facilitas' meaning 'easiness', and the verb 'to facilitate' means 'to make easy, promote or help forward'. From this it can be suggested that 'facilitation' describes the process of enabling students to learn and to adapt or change their behaviour by:

- providing a helping hand
- removing obstacles
- creating a smooth pathway for the students to pursue their learning journey.

Facilitation is a style of teaching that is fundamental to work-based learning and stems from the work of the psychologist Carl Rogers. He developed ideas in understanding how students learn most effectively, including student-centred learning which is non-critical, non-directive, self-directed and reflective and where students are involved in the learning process (Sharp *et al.* 2010). The difference between teaching and facilitating learning is that facilitators concentrate on providing the resources and opportunities for learning to take place, rather than managing and controlling learning. The facilitator is neither a 'content expert' nor a lecturer.

Effective facilitation involves the following steps:

- Prepare:
  - Set the initial mood or climate.
  - Help identify students' needs.
  - Organise and make accessible a wide range of resources for learning.
  - Be aware of the students' learning style, but help the students to work outside the confines of their chosen learning style.
- Be clear of your role as a facilitator:
  - Keep the student focused on the task and process.
  - Encourage participation, but remember that individuals participate in different ways. Some may talk very little, but they are still participating.
  - Others may wish to talk constantly and may be contributing little.
  - Help make connections.
  - Share opinions. Do so in ways that do not demand or impose but represent simply a personal sharing which students may take or leave.

- Do not do the work for the student. Learning is more effective and lasting if the individuals discover on their own (learning by doing).
- Spend time ensuring that the student grasps the tasks and concepts.
- Recognise and accept your own limitations.
- Relax.
- Adopt a facilitative approach:
  - Listen more than talk.
  - Frequently ask if there are questions. When you ask a question, allow time for students to think before answering.
  - Be sensitive to gender and culture.
  - Encourage critical thinking.
  - Remain as objective as possible.
  - Be alert to signs of confusion and review tasks that are causing confusion.
  - Do not feel you must be an expert. Remind the students and yourself that you are a facilitator, and use their expertise and experience.
  - Ask another student for their ideas on a question; do not feel you have to answer it yourself.
  - Be flexible. Keep depth and breadth of content flexible. Changing something does not mean you planned poorly, but probably means you are listening, watching and adjusting your plans to fit the situation.

In conclusion, the work-based facilitator needs to utilise a range of skills in their facilitatory role to ensure effective placement learning. Intrinsic feedback acquired through reflection on the role is a useful aid for facilitators to know how effective they are at supporting learning in the workplace (the unit on reflection will inform that approach to evaluating the role). However, work-based facilitators also need external feedback to inform development of the role. The next section of this unit will consider external approaches to evaluating the role.

ACTIVITY 2.13

Can you give an example of facilitation as part of your role in supporting learning and assessment in your workplace?

How effective were your skills in facilitation? Identify specific strengths and areas that require development.

Tips for effective supervision

- maintain regular contact with the student
- be honest at all times
- avoid being judgemental
- recognise that you also need support
- don't expect to have all answers
- help students to access resources and additional support
- make your expectations and boundaries clear to the student
- work with the student on his/her difficulties
- maintain confidentiality.

Tips for students to ensure effective learning

- accept challenges willingly
- share your feelings about how the relationship with the facilitator is working
- be positive

- take an active role in own learning
- trust the facilitator
- be prepared to discuss issues openly
- recognise the need to take risks to progress
- identify ways of self development outside the relationship with the facilitator
- don't expect too much of the facilitator
- talk about the end of the relationship as it approaches.

Evaluating the facilitator in supporting learning in the workplace

Congdon *et al.* (2010) identify two key questions on any evaluation of a student's workplace experience:

- What would you do the same?
- What would you change?

The Quality Assurance Agency (2010) believes that evaluation of a workplace learning environment should include the following features:

- review of student progress
- use of feedback from facilitators and students
- establishment of procedures within which feedback on the quality and standards of the placement can be received and appropriate action taken where necessary
- formal and informal means of gathering feedback.

Behaviours that can help facilitate the evaluation process include careful monitoring, regulation and decision-making, open communication, willingness to offer explanations and justifications, evaluation of alternatives, planning and inferring (Hine 2012). The frequency of evaluation and the method of assessment should be addressed at the time the workplace learning opportunity is first structured. Ideally, student supervision should be part of the facilitator's job description and valued as an investment in the future. It should not create conflict with the facilitator's role as an employee in the workplace.

The focus of the evaluation should be on the characteristics that students perceive as valuable and helpful in a facilitator, including:

- An envisioner who is enthusiastic about opportunities or possibilities and inspires interest.
- An energiser who makes the subject fascinating, and is enthusiastic and dynamic.
- A role model whom the student can look up to, values and admires and may wish to emulate.
- An investor who spends a lot of time with the student, spots potential and capabilities, and who can hand over responsibility.
- A supporter who is willing to listen and is warm and caring and available in times of need.
- An eye-opener who inspires interest in research and is able to facilitate understanding of wider issues.
- A door-opener, who includes the student in discussions, asks the student to be a representative on committees and delegates a range of tasks to the learner.
- A problem-solver, helping the student to figure out and try out new ideas, who can analyse strengths and create ways to use them.

A facilitator may want to focus on their role as a student's assessor by considering their effectiveness as:

- A feedback-giver who can offer both positive and negative reaction feedback and help the student to examine the things that go wrong.
- A challenger who questions opinions and beliefs, and forces the learner to examine decisions.

- A teacher-coach who can instruct about setting priorities, help develop interpersonal skills, give guidance on workplace tasks and encourage the student to gain from experience.
- An idea-booster who not only discusses issues, problems and goals, but also allows the student to present and argue ideas.
- A standard prodder who is very clear about what level of performance is required and pushes and prods the student to achieve it.

Facilitators might also want to evaluate their role in delivering presentations to students. Carlton College (2009) outlines a structure for evaluating presentations:

- Subject: Was the presentation informative? Did it have a clear focus? Was it well researched?
- Organization/clarity: Was it easy to follow? Was there a clear introduction and conclusion?
- Preparation: Had the speaker rehearsed? Was s/he in control of the sequence, pacing and flow of the presentation? Did s/he make effective use of notes, without relying on them too heavily?
- Sensitivity to audience: Did the speaker maintain eye contact with all members of the class? Did s/he give you time to take notes as needed? Did s/he repeat the main ideas more than once? Did s/he make effective use of pauses, gestures, change in pace and pitch?
- Visual aids: Did the speaker make effective use of handouts, overheads and/or the whiteboard? Were overheads or board writing large enough to see easily?

Rae (2010) sets out a series of questions that could be used to inform the content of a placement evaluation questionnaire. Potential questions include:

- To what extent do you feel you have learned from the placement?
- To what extent do you feel you have had previous learning (perhaps some you have forgotten) confirmed?
- What have you NOT learned that you needed to and /or expected to learn during the placement? Please describe fully any items.
- To what extent have you developed your behavioural skills?
- To what extent do you feel your personal learning objectives have been achieved?
- Which of your personal objectives were not achieved, and why?
- Which parts of the placement do you feel were most useful?
- Which parts of the placement do you feel were least useful, or not at all useful?
- What other topics would you have liked to be included in the placement?
- To make way for any additional material, what would you omit from the placement?
- How would you rate the placement overall?
- To what extent have the objectives of the programme been achieved?
- To what extent have your personal objectives for attending the placement been achieved?
- To what extent has your understanding of the subject improved or increased as a result of the placement?
- To what extent have your skills in the subject improved or increased as a result of the placement?
- To what extent has the placement helped to enhance your appreciation and understanding of the subject?
- What is your overall rating of the placement?
- To what extent would you recommend others with similar needs to your own to use this placement?
- To what extent was material necessary to the placement provided to you prior to the placement?

Evaluation results should be shared with relevant partners, e.g. work colleagues, higher education institution. Once the evaluation method and schedule has been identified, a plan to review the evaluations should be discussed in order to continue and strengthen what works, and to address and revise what doesn't work. Regular evaluation and continuous improvement can

References

Burrill. J., Hussain, Z., Prescott, D. and Waywell, L. (2010) *An Introduction to Practice Education.* www.science.ulster.ac.uk/nursing/mentorship/learning_materials.php

Carlton College (2009) *Planning Student Presentations.* http://serc.carleton.edu/introgeo/campusbased/presentation.html

Clark, D. (2010) *Communication and Leadership.* www.nwlink.com/~donclark/leader/leadcom.html.

Congdon, G., Wakins, G., Baker, T., Stewart, H., Thompson, E., Keenan, C. and Gibson, J. (2010) *Managing the Placement Learning Environment.* www.science.ulster.ac.uk/nursing/mentorship/learning_materials.php

Conneticut Learns (2012) *Workplace Mentoring Guide.* www.sde.ct.gov/sde/lib/sde/PDF/DEPS/Career/WB/mentoring.pdf

Cortright, S. M. (2012) *10 Tips to Effective and Active Listening Skills.* http://powertochange.com/students/people/listen

Gray, M. and Smith, L. (2000) The Qualities of an Effective Mentor from the Student Nurse's Perspective: Findings from a Longitudinal Qualitative Study. *Journal of Advanced Nursing* 32(6):1542–1549.

Hine, A. (2012) *Mirroring Effective Education through Mentoring, Metacognition and Self Reflection.* www.aare.edu.au/00pap/hin00017.htm

Kleffner, J. H. and Hendrickson, W. D. (2001) *Effective Clinical Teaching.* www.utexas.edu/pharmacy/general/experiential/practitioner/effectiveprec.pdf

Leading Insight (2012) *Giving Effective Feedback.* www.leadinginsight.com/ezine_feedback.htm

Management Sciences for Health (2012) *Negotiation Techniques.* http://erc.msh.org/quality/ittools/itnegot2.cfm

Middlesex University (2010) *The Four Cornerstones of an Affective Learning Environment.* http://hsscplacements.middlesex.wikispaces.net/file/detail/The+Four+Cornerstones+of+an+Effective+Learning+Environment.doc.

Quality Assurance Agency (2010) *Code of Practice for the Assurance of Academic Quality and Standards in Higher Education: Placement learning.* www.qaa.ac.uk/Publications/InformationAndGuidance/Pages/Code-of-practice-Section-9.aspx

Rae, L. (2010) *Training Programme Evaluation.* www.businessballs.com/trainingprogramevaluation.htm

Ramaley, J. A. (2009) *The Seven Principles for Good Practice.* www.winona.edu/faculty/478.asp

Sharp, P., Ainslie, T., Hamphill, A., Hobson, S., Merriman, C., Ong, P. and Roche, J. (2010) *Mentoring.* www.science.ulster.ac.uk/nursing/mentorship/learning_materials.php

Sisco, B. R. (1991) Setting the Climate for Effective Teaching and Learning. In Hiemstra R, *Creating Effective Environments for Effective Adult Learning.* Jossey-Bass.

University of Newcastle-upon-Tyne (2009) *Communicating Skills: Making Oral Presentations.* http://lorien.ncl.ac.uk/ming/dept/tips/present/comms.htm

Wang, C. M. and Ong, G. (2003) *Questioning Techniques for Active Learning.* www.cdtl.nus.edu.sg/Ideas/iot2.htm

Reflection on and in the workplace

Introduction

Reflection involves describing, analysing and evaluating our thoughts, assumptions, beliefs, theories and actions (Fade 2012). Since the aim of placement is to promote 'Clinical reasoning and analytical and evaluation abilities in students' (McClure 2012), reflection is central to development of reflective practice. It is assumed that reflection is a process that is engaged in as part of learning; however, reflection is a skill which needs to be developed and enhanced.

Aim of unit

This unit aims to identify the importance of reflection in teaching and learning and to discuss how it might be used in the workplace. The different models of reflection will be considered, as well as how you can assist the learner in reflecting upon their practice/work and learning whilst at the same time enhancing your own reflective skills.

Outcomes of unit

At the end of this unit of learning you will be able to:

1 discuss the use of reflection in learning
2 identify barriers to reflection and ways to minimise their effects
3 use a model of reflection to facilitate student learning in the workplace
4 facilitate a process where the learner reflects critically on their practice/work.

What is reflection?

The image of looking at oneself in a mirror, suggested by the word, means that it has implications of being conscious of what one is doing. Because of this it is a word that is widely used but not always understood. Rowntree (1992), for example, praises the reflective student who thinks about her own experience of studying and decides what changes of approach might be most suitable.

Rowntree (1992) says that reflection is studying one's own study methods as seriously as one studies the subject and thinking about a learning task after you have done it. Unless you do this, he says, the task will almost certainly be wasted.

In any learning situation, he says, you should prepare for it beforehand, participate actively during it, and reflect on it afterwards.

He applies these points to working in small groups, suggesting note-taking in the group as an aid to reflection afterwards, and also suggesting reflection on how the group operates. It is important, therefore, that reflection is on what is happening in the workplace and why the learning is different or unique because it is happening in the workplace.

ACTIVITY 3.1

It is important before teaching others that you have some understanding of your own learning styles and how you reflect upon events. This activity assists you in this process.

How do you reflect on your current professional practice?

Can you give three examples of how reflection has led to changes and improvements in your professional practice?

How could you further develop your reflection style?

Types of reflection

Schön (1987) in his work identifies two types of reflection: reflection-in-action (thinking on your feet) and reflection-on-action (retrospective thinking). He suggests that reflection is used by practitioners when they encounter situations that are unique, and when individuals may not be able to apply known theories or techniques previously learnt through formal education.

Definitions of reflection

Dewey (2009) defined reflection as: an active persistent and careful consideration of any belief or supposed form of knowledge in the light of the grounds that support it and the further conclusion to which it tends.

Boud *et al.* (2006) take a different perspective and define it as a generic term for those intellectual and effective activities in which individuals engage to explore their experiences in order to lead to a new understanding and appreciation. They view reflection from the learner's point of view. They discuss the relationship of the reflective process and the learning experience against what the learner can do.

Reid (1993) in her definition also noted reflection as an active process rather than passive thinking. She states: 'Reflection is a process of reviewing an experience of practice in order to describe, analyse, evaluate and so inform learning about practice.'

Kemmis (1985) agrees with Reid that the process of reflection is more than a process that focuses 'on the head'. It is, he argues, a positive active process that reviews, analyses and evaluates experiences, draws on theoretical concepts or previous learning and so provides an action plan for future experiences.

Johns (2005) notes that reflection enables the practitioner to assess, understand and learn through their experiences. It is a personal process that usually results in some change for the individual in their perspective of a situation or creates new learning for the individual.

Reflection starts with the individual or group and their own experiences and can result, if applied to practice, in improvement of the clinical skills performed by the individual through new knowledge gained on reflection. This process of reflection, if then related into practice, can assist the individual in gaining the required knowledge, leading to a potential improvement in the quality of the care received from that individual. The outcome of reflection as identified by Mezirow (1981) is learning. Louden (1991) describes in ordinary language reflection as serious and sober thought at some distance from action and which has connotations similar to 'meditation' and 'introspection'. It is a mental process that takes place out of the stream of action, looking forward or (usually) back to actions that have taken place.

Reflection and professional learning

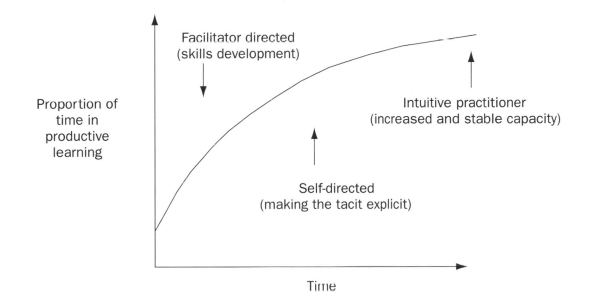

Figure 3.1 Increasing capacity as self-directed reflective practitioner (adapted from Stephen Powell 2004)

Critically reflective learning is nurtured by relationships between teacher and learner, learner and learner, and both of these and the subject under study. Powell (2005) identified the optimal relationship, indicated in Figure 3.1, as mutual, open, challenging, contextually aware and characterised by dialogue (Brockbank and McGill 1998).

Becoming a reflective practitioner/worker

According to the educator Boud *et al.* (2006), effective learning will not occur unless you reflect. To do this, you must think of a particular moment in time, ponder over it and go back through it, and only then will you gain new insights into different aspects of that situation. According to Kolb (1984) reflecting is an essential element of learning. This is shown through an experiential learning cycle illustrated in Figure 3.2.

McClure (2012) suggests that, if you follow this cycle in a clockwise direction with your student, you will see that after having had an experience the student has to reflect on what he/she saw or did, by reviewing the whole situation in his/her mind. This may be assisted by looking at it on film, discussing it with others, thinking abstractly about the event for a while, or seeking advice or further information.

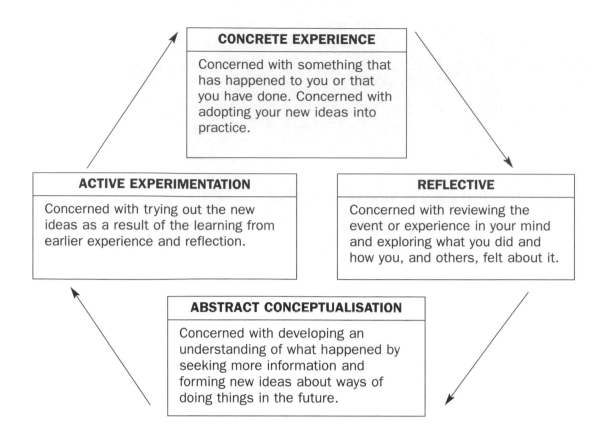

CONCRETE EXPERIENCE

Concerned with something that has happened to you or that you have done. Concerned with adopting your new ideas into practice.

ACTIVE EXPERIMENTATION

Concerned with trying out the new ideas as a result of the learning from earlier experience and reflection.

REFLECTIVE

Concerned with reviewing the event or experience in your mind and exploring what you did and how you, and others, felt about it.

ABSTRACT CONCEPTUALISATION

Concerned with developing an understanding of what happened by seeking more information and forming new ideas about ways of doing things in the future.

Figure 3.2 Kolb's learning cycle (adapted from Kolb 1984)

Eventually the student will probably come up with ideas for approaching the situation differently next time. He/she will then try out their ideas to see if they are effective. He/she will thus complete the learning cycle and start over again with a view to refining his/her actions. This is an on-going process, so we will never achieve perfection. We will always find other ways of doing things based on our learning from previous experiences.

Building up experience is a gradual process. The student will develop reflective abilities during the course of their learning on placement. Reflection should initially develop in safe environments where mistakes are tolerated. He/she can then reflect and discuss the decisions that were made during their supervision sessions with their work-based facilitator. Reflection should become integral to these sessions.

When reflecting-on-action, the first step in the process is the description of the incident, and it is advisable that student health care practitioners keep a reflective diary, as memory cannot be relied upon for the detail of events, in which they record details of incidents that either troubled or pleased them, recording details as soon after the event as possible.

Much attention has been given to the value of recording events and experiences in written form, particularly through the use of reflective diaries and journals (Chimera 2007). The exercise of diary writing promotes both the qualities required for reflection, i.e. open-mindedness and motivation, as well as the skills, i.e. self-awareness; description and observation; critical analysis and problem-solving; and synthesis and evaluation (Richardson and Maltby 1995).

Time for reflection

McClure (2012) continues to identify how important the time for reflection is. The work-based facilitator must make time for reflection so that it becomes part of your and the students' way of working. Reflection is an integral part of practice and students need time to develop this skill.

It is not a process that can be rushed, but neither is it a process that has to occur at a particular time. Thus, the student can reflect on his/her journey to and from placement, or between activities or during lunch break. It is a good idea to encourage the student to sum up each day with a reflective comment in his/her diary, spending only a few minutes doing it. If the student knows that you expect them to reflect on their practice in this structured way, they will be more likely to keep and benefit from their reflective diary. You may also set them an example by keeping a reflective diary of your own professional practice or indeed your experiences as a work-based facilitator, thus demonstrating that learning is always on-going!

Keeping a reflective diary

Each individual will have a different way of keeping a reflective diary. There are, however, some general points to reinforce to learners about their diary.

It should be:

- a record that is useful to you
- a cue to memory
- honestly written
- enjoyable to you in its production.

It can be used:

- to describe key events in your practice
- to evaluate key events in your practice
- to engage in focused evaluation of recurring themes
- to reflect on what may have become habitual
- to develop and appraise action taken.

Getting started:

- Set aside time for writing.
- Allow time for the sifting of thoughts and ideas.
- Do not worry about style, presentation.
- Remember that the aim is to facilitate reflection on practice.
- Find evidence to back up your thoughts: what evidence do I have for what I have just written?

Begin by asking:

- How do I see my role as a student on workplace placement (purposes and intentions)?
- Why did I become a student?
- What kind of practitioner do I think I am?
- What values do I believe in?
- How do I demonstrate that I am practising in a way that is consistent with relevant professional values and codes of conduct?

Reflective questions

The following is a set of questions that could be used to assist your thinking, perhaps when you are writing up your reflections on practice in a diary or when you are thinking back over an experience and discussing it with your work-based facilitator.

- What was I aiming for when I did that?
- What exactly did I do? How would I describe it precisely?
- Why did I choose that particular action?

- What theories/models/research informed my actions?
- What was I trying to achieve?
- What did I do next?
- What were the reasons for doing that?
- How successful was it?
- What criteria am I using to judge success?
- What alternatives were there?
- Could I have dealt with the situation any better?
- How would I do it differently next time?
- What do I feel about the whole experience?
- What knowledge/values/skills were demonstrated?
- How did the client feel about it?
- How do I know the client felt like that?
- What sense can I make of this in the light of my past experience?
- Has this changed the way in which I will do things in the future?

A final note

Reflective diaries are a private record of experiences throughout placement and so it is important to use them to report thoughts, feelings and opinions rather than merely the factual events of the day. Only by reporting personal feelings following an event can experiences be built upon and improved.

It is important to use the reflective diary to record positive experiences and achievements as well as the not-so-positive ones. A balanced view of what has taken place is essential.

Reflective diaries are not just important during placement – I kept my reflective diary and think of it to be, to some extent, rather like a personal 'Record of Achievement'.

ACTIVITY 3.3

Having considered the need for reflection and the methods available to assist in this, undertake the following activity to explore how you can use reflection in students' learning in the workplace.

What methods would you use to ensure students were discussing their reflections with you?

Effective reflection supervision and assessment in the workplace

Reflection is not an 'add-on' piece to your learning process, portfolio, or teaching practice. It is integral to the complex process of becoming an educator. Successful reflection enables self-awareness, personal and professional growth and improved teaching practices.

Reflection may be accomplished individually and collectively. You will have opportunities to reflect on your experiences and teaching with others, such as peers, other mentors, facilitators and university lecturers. Each will bring a unique perspective to your understanding of yourself developing as an effective work-based facilitator.

Ultimately, self-reflection and dialogue with others will result in insights as to:

1 how and why you think the way you do about teaching, learning and assessment
2 what actions you took, what choices you made
3 the meaning of your actions and choices
4 what learning and growth has occurred
5 how you can change your practices in the future
6 what you believe is the social value of education
7 what you believe is your role as a professional and educator.

What is the purpose of reflection?

Dewey (2009) stated that reflection thus implies that something is believed in (or disbelieved in), not on its own direct account, but through something else that stands as witness, evidence, proof, voucher or warrant; that is, as ground of belief. For Dewey, reflective thinking consisted of two parts: a state of doubt and a search to resolve that doubt. Thus, constructing a portfolio is an act of revealing one's beliefs. Schön (1987) considered there to be a utility for reflective thinking in that cognitive practice has a direct relationship to practices within professional realms (teaching). At the heart of portfolio development is purposeful choice making. The portfolio development process is organic.

Your portfolio can be entered into again and again with new reflections that can provide new insights.

Where do you put the reflections in your portfolio?

Your portfolio is an assessment portfolio. This means that it includes a collection of selected artefacts and focused reflections and goals that demonstrate how you have met the learning outcomes. Reflections should be infused throughout your portfolio.

What makes good evidence?

The search for evidence is a quest for quality. The reflection process will assist you to determine how evidence is collected and presented. Evidence selection requires that you place value upon an experience or event. As you develop your portfolio, you will be gathering evidence that demonstrates your competencies in each of the Standards 1–8. A good piece of evidence is:

- carefully selected
- representative of the standard
- a demonstration of your competencies of the standard
- presented professionally
- personally meaningful
- paired with a relevant and insightful reflection (reflections can be written, audio or video-taped).

> **ACTIVITY 3.4**
>
> Evidence is an essential part of the reflective process. This activity asks you to look at the following:
>
> What evidence would you select/use to demonstrate your competence and development as a workplace facilitator?
>
> What do you think would best demonstrate students' learning in your workplace?

Learning through and from reflection

If the student can be 'coached' to identify the thought processes undergone to move from ignorance to understanding – to reflect on his or her own learning – then learning can continue at a much swifter pace and with less support from the mentor/educator.

For a minority of lecturers, the label says it all. Their self-image is of a subject expert whose main task is to deliver knowledge and then to test whether the message has been properly received and understood. Learning is assumed to be happening despite the clear evidence to the contrary.

Mentoring and reflective practice

Gillings (2000) states that commitment to self-enquiry and a readiness to change practice are important if the individual is to get the most out of the process.

Many authors identify self-awareness as essential to the reflective process. This implies that the individual needs to be well informed/appraised of his/her own character, including beliefs and values. Many models of reflective practice also include self-awareness and questioning of beliefs, values and attitudes.

The last stage of many models of reflection relates to a willingness to change practice, where new conceptual perspectives are reached in order to inform practice. If the learner is not willing to change practice he/she will not gain the potential benefits from the process in terms of practice development, advances will not be made and professional practice will not evolve.

Many of the skills identified as essential for a good facilitator are required by the work-based facilitator to guide the reflective practitioner. A willingness to commit time to the process and to listen to the learner helps foster a relationship that can bring challenging issues to the fore.

There are many similarities between reflective practice and supervision. Therefore, learners can make effective use of reflective practice as a learning tool within the context of supervision. It is, however, important that the learner and the work-based facilitator are committed to the process and have a shared understanding of the process to make the experience effective (McClure 2012).

Supervision

Supervision can be both formal and informal. Informal feedback is given regularly and constructively in a non-judgemental way. Formal supervision should occur regularly at prearranged times in a quiet environment free from the distractions of service delivery. Supervision sessions should last about one hour and form an essential feature of the placement and facilitatory process. Alsop and Ryan (1999) state that formal supervision should be used for four main purposes:

1   reflection, feedback on and dialogue about practice
2   review of the achievement of learning goals
3   revision of the learning contract, until the next supervision session
4   exploration of practice issues to a deeper level of understanding.

Therefore, formal supervision is a time for exploring practice, a time for learning, where the real objective is facilitating the student's growth. Work-based facilitators must therefore ensure that they acknowledge the importance of these sessions and allocate appropriate time for them.

Both the work-based facilitator and the student need to prepare well for the formal supervision sessions. The student needs to be encouraged to think through selected experiences, reviewing them in his/her mind, so that he/she learns from what happened. The work-based facilitator may guide the discussion, prompting the student and probing his/her knowledge and understanding, but essentially the student must do the work. This must then be recorded in the relevant form.

Learning from significant events

Each of us in our professional lives is likely to face a variety of critical incidents during which an ethical dilemma arises. Often we handle such dilemmas by reacting based on our past experiences, our emotional health at the time and/or 'what seems to be right'. However, it is possible to be proactive, rather than reactive, and use an ethical decision-making process to guide your responses. The purpose of this section is to show how this might work.

Brockett/Hiemstra ethics decision-making process

Brockett and Hiemstra (1991) have developed an ethics decision-making process that can be used for critical incident sorting and analysis. We believe it provides the kind of information needed to help you make appropriate ethical decisions. Once you get used to the process and have it incorporated as part of your professional skills, such decisions can become automatic for many of the incidents you will face. Thus, whenever you are faced with some sort of actual or potential ethical dilemma, we suggest you consider an interaction of your personal values with the obligations you have to others and consider the consequences of any actions in light of these values and obligations.

For example, the following questions might be helpful groundings for your personal values:

1   What do I believe about human nature, the education of adults, and about ethics?
2   How committed am I to these beliefs that I hold?
3   Which basic values actually drive my practice as a professional adult educator?

In terms of personal obligations, ask yourself such questions as these:

1   To whom am I responsible?
2   To what extent is the dilemma I am facing a result of conflicting obligations (this often will be the case)?

Then consider the consequences of any of your actions:

1   What are my options?
2   What are possible consequences of my actions?
3   Which option is most consistent with my values?

Obviously, some actions or decisions must be made on the spot and time for the kind of critical reflection we are suggesting will be limited. However, whenever it is possible we suggest taking your decision-making process through a more deliberate process like the one described above. We believe that not only will you be more likely to stay consistent with your ethical dimensions of practice, but you also will begin to incorporate such a decision-making framework within your daily practice. Subsequently, ethical decision-making will come easier and quicker for you. The following incident illustrates how this can occur.

A simulated critical incident

As a brand new Assistant Professor, Dr Smith realised that publish or perish was a very real characteristic of his institution. His Department Chair had explained clearly the importance of scholarship as well as good teaching and service to his university, community, and profession. Thus, he set about building a research agenda, establishing a regular schedule for research and writing, and learning from his experienced colleagues.

Thus, he was flattered when at the end of his first year he was approached by one of the Senior Professors in the College and asked if he would be interested in co-authoring some research articles. He and the senior professor then established a research project, collected and analysed some appropriate data, and began the process of writing two articles. Dr Smith agreed to be the junior author on such articles and the writing efforts were fairly equally shared.

The senior professor undertook the responsibility of finding a journal for the two articles and he handled all the communications. He happily reported back to Dr Smith within a few weeks that a journal had agreed to publish both articles in a special issue on adult education. Approximately six months later Dr Smith received from the senior professor a couple of copies of the journal containing the two articles. Overall it had been a good learning experience. It had helped enhance Dr Smith's reputation within the College and increased his confidence, and was an important step in the movement toward eventual promotion.

Unfortunately, the story did not end at that happy juncture. At the end of that year, Dr Smith received in the mail from the publisher a letter thanking him for his contributions to the journal that year and his personal wishes that the income from the efforts would be useful in helping fund future research. Dr Smith called the publisher for clarification and was told that the senior professor had been sent a cheque for a certain sum of money and he had told the publisher that he would take out money to cover incurred expenses and then send a cheque to Dr Smith.

This created a real ethical dilemma for Dr Smith. Without much thought, he confronted the senior professor and demanded to know what had happened. The senior professor quickly explained that he had forgotten to send Dr Smith a cheque and promptly wrote one out. However, because others were in the office when this happened, it was an embarrassing situation and a real professional distance was created that lasted throughout the time that Dr Smith was at that university. Unfortunately, no additional co-authoring between these two individuals took place.

Could Dr Smith have handled it differently? What were the long-term ramifications?

Critical incident sorting and analysis

Dr Smith did not go through any sort of decision-making process. Out of personal anger, and perhaps arrogance, he publicly confronted the senior professor without discussing various possibilities or explanations. This resulted in public embarrassment for the senior professor, a lost opportunity to find out what was the real story and the creation of a distance that may have been, in the long run, detrimental to Dr Smith and the adult education profession. Certainly, there is the possibility that the senior professor purposely overlooked making the payment, but it was never possible to determine that fact.

Personal values sorting was possible for Dr Smith if he had asked some of the following questions:

1. What do I believe about human nature, the education of adults, and about ethics?
   - I have a basic trust in others.
   - There is real value in making any sort of a contribution to the education of adults.
   - I have a basic belief in professional honesty.
2. How committed am I to the beliefs that I hold?
   - Each of these beliefs should be a central core for my actions.
   - I must constantly work to uphold these beliefs.
   - I also have a need to believe that others share in some of these basic beliefs.
3. Which basic values actually drive my practice as a professional adult educator?
   - I value humanistic beliefs and a notion that the dignity of each human being must be respected – these serve as a foundation for what I do as a professional.
   - I try hard to be consistent not only in what I do as a professional but also in my role as spouse, parent, friend, and community member.
   - The reality that I embrace rests on an assumption that all humans are basically good and have potential for continuous growth and development as individuals.

Personal obligation sorting would lead to the following questions:

1. To whom am I responsible?
   - I am responsible not only for myself, but also for what my actions might do in terms of relationships with others.
   - I also have a responsibility to ensure that good research and scholarship results in accurate and useful information being disseminated to practitioners and other researchers.
2. To what extent was the dilemma I faced a result of conflicting obligations?
   - I had an obligation to protect the income my family received.
   - I had an obligation to protect the reputation of the senior professor, if possible.
   - I had an obligation to stay true to my humanistic values and beliefs.

3   What were the possible consequences of the actions I took (or might have taken)?
   • My options could have included discussing the situation with the senior professor behind closed doors to find out what really happened.
   • Another option could have been to simply forget the whole situation because of the value I received from the experience, the counsel and support from the senior professor, and the knowledge that I had contributed information about adult education to a population of readers who otherwise might not have received the information.
   • One real consequence was the fact that I never again had an opportunity to work with this professor (and some of his close colleagues).
   • Another consequence was that my public confrontation no doubt raised questions in the minds of others about me and that senior professor.
   • The very first option noted above would have been most consistent with my values and might have resulted in a clearer understanding of what happened plus future co-authoring opportunities that could have further benefited many audiences.

ACTIVITY 3.5

Think of a recent dilemma you have had to deal with whilst supporting a student. Use the decision-making process model to analyse how you dealt with this dilemma. (This may be useful to include in your portfolio.)

Tools for reflection

Reflective thinking is a multifaceted process. It is an analysis of events and circumstances. By virtue of its complexity, the task of teaching requires constant and continual observation, evaluation and subsequent action. However, to be an effective work-based facilitator, it is not enough to be able to recognise what happens in the workplace. Rather, it is imperative to understand the 'whys', 'hows', and 'what ifs' as well. This understanding comes through the consistent practice of reflective thinking.

Reflective thinking is a learned process that requires time. Generally there is little, if any, time left at the day's end to reflect on previous events and to design meaningful, creative, problem-solving strategies. However, given the intent of the student teaching experience, time for reflection should be a critical and on-going practice. The following are some examples of activities that promote reflection and may be tailored to fit into the working day and beyond.

Thinking aloud: Intentionally express out loud thinking about your learning. This is especially effective when teaching the student how to plan. It uncovers the reasoning behind making decisions. Another component of thinking aloud is describing and analysing positive and negative experiences as they surface. This can be a therapeutic and valuable tool that can be accomplished alone or in conjunction with individuals from the mentoring team.

Reflective journal: This is a process of recording and analysing events in a prescribed manner, which can be a productive strategy to foster reflective thinking. The journal process may be formal or informal. It can be a description of a significant event or an aspect of learning on which a student is asked to focus.

Competency continuum: Think about the areas in teaching identified in the student's learning outcomes. Begin by identifying the factors that inhibit the student's ability to be more competent and identify what would be most helpful to gain more competencies. Use this continuum as a tool for discussion and action planning between you and your student.

Data collection/action research: Consider a problem area such as student motivation that concerns you. Intentionally design a procedure for collecting information (data) to learn more about the problem. Use this data to further analyse the situation, to act on the problem, or to re-evaluate.

Video/audio tape and reflective analysis: Video or audio tape your teaching. View or listen to the tape for the purpose of analysing your instruction and student response. The video or audio tape may be used as a tool for reflective dialogue between the student and you. It could be combined with a journal entry.

Written self-evaluation: This is a structured self-analysis.

Use of the problem-solving process: This six-step process may be used for any problem situation in or out of the classroom setting. It is intended as a tool for collaborative or individual problem-solving and reflective thinking as well as a design for action.

1   Identify the problem.
2   Generate possible solutions.
3   Evaluate the solutions.
4   Design an action plan.
5   Implement the plan.
6   Evaluate the results.

Coaching and conferencing process: This is a process that occurs on a regular basis during the student teaching experience. It provides an opportunity to talk about teaching and learning and should be a natural flow of conversation that includes sharing ideas and giving and receiving formative feedback. This process may be on-going and informal, or scheduled and structured. It may or may not include an observation. The intent of the process is to engage in an activity that promotes dialogue about teaching effectiveness, and encourages reflective thinking about teaching, learning, and performance.

Development of a professional portfolio: The process of creating and selecting documents for inclusion in the portfolio requires a significant amount of reflective thinking about yourself as a teacher and your growth related to the performance standards for student teaching. It is an opportunity to talk about your experience and performance with the individuals who form your mentoring team. It can be one of the most intensive processes for reflection.

Individual reflection

The presence of others can support individual learning in many ways, but it is also good to provide individuals with some personal time and space to reflect – away from the distractions of others. However, being alone is no guarantee of high quality reflection: when alone, attention can wander or people get stuck in a rut as they keep going through the same patterns of thought or visiting the same dead ends. But find the right setting or technique for individual reflection and you can help people see with fresh eyes, or lead them to 'aha' moments, or help them break out of 'same-old' thinking. Here are just some options for 'reviewing for one':

*   unstructured reflective writing: using log books, diaries, journals, notebooks
*   structured reflective writing: responding to a questionnaire or to a standard template of questions or headings following a particular sequence
*   graphic reflection techniques: creating diagrams, charts, graphs, maps, patterns, drawings, collages or photos to capture reflections
*   scavenger hunt: searching for symbolic objects that answer reflective questions
*   solo time: time alone without distractions and with space to think, or to read feedback notes from other group members, or as a challenge in itself – to live alone and close to nature with time to reflect
*   guided reflection: listening to a monologue that includes pauses for thought
*   silence: context is all-important, but use of well-timed silences in suitable settings can result in deep reflection
*   reflection time: following a stimulating story, performance or experience
*   thinking time: before making a reflective statement about recent events
*   preparation time: before making a presentation about personal learning to the group.

Some of the above individual reviewing techniques can work surprisingly well, but often the best way to make a breakthrough is reviewing with another person, for example a colleague.

Reviewing for two: roles for reviewing in pairs

Talking things through with another person can be more dynamic and productive than being left with your own thoughts. Sometimes the other person is just a listener, but there are many other useful roles the other person can adopt – such as a sounding board, a summariser, a buddy, a coach, or even a devil's advocate. There is no guarantee that the other person will be good at assisting the process of reflection. The other person may be too intrusive or challenging, or may stumble into 'no-go' areas, or offer insensitive advice. There is always the risk that the other person (even a skilled facilitator) will spoil, distort or disrupt the process of reflection. The risk of ending up with an 'unhelpful' listener can be reduced by providing clear briefings and by providing an easy way for the 'speaker' to change the rules or opt out if they find the process is not working well.

Here are a few helpful roles that the 'other person' can play when reviewing in pairs:

- Listener: just listens – giving the 'reflector' the opportunity to think aloud.
- Sounding board: listens and responds to any questions that the reflector may ask.
- Summariser: repeats key phrases, summarises, asks for clarification.
- Buddy: notices, empathises, supports, and possibly advises.
- Coach: agrees objectives, provides feedback, and asks questions that assist reflection.
- Interviewer (with a script): asks set questions or follows a certain review sequence.
- Child: just keeps asking 'why?'. The reflector can stop the process at any point.
- Devil's advocate: tests and challenges what the reflector says. This needs careful briefing to ensure that the challenges are provided and perceived as being part of a helpful process.

Reviewing for two: walking and talking

Something that goes particularly well with paired reviews is 'walking and talking', especially if you have a suitable outdoor location. 'Walking and talking' can be combined with any of the above roles. A classic problem in paired reviews is that one person dominates and the time is not well shared. One solution is to divide the total time into two halves by having a clear 'swap-over point' at half way (see 'Out and back'). Another solution is to have a turn-taking system in which there is frequent swapping of roles (see 'Chat cards'). These and other variations of 'walking and talking' are described next:

- Out and back: this helps to ensure that the time is divided equally between each person. Pairs walk out to an agreed point, swap roles and walk back in their new roles. (See previous section for ideas about 'roles'.) Ideally, each pair heads for a different point to avoid distractions from other pairs.
- Chat cards: each card has a reflective question. Each person takes it in turns to answer as they walk. One question per card helps people to focus on one question at a time. Just one good question may be enough for some pairs, but other pairs may need a plentiful supply of questions to keep a reflective conversation going. It is better to have too many questions than too few.
- Scavenger hunt: pairs work together to collect symbolic objects that answer reflective questions.
- Walking round the active reviewing cycle: as pairs walk through each stage of the cycle, they focus their reflective conversation on the stage they are walking through. In practice this takes two or three minutes in each stage, so you either need a huge cycle or people simply stop and talk until they are ready to move on to the next stage.

Reviewing for two: changing partners

Another style of paired review is where people have a series of brief meetings with different partners. The speed of this process means that people do not get stuck in partnerships that are not working. There may not be very deep reflection during brief meetings, but a quick succession of paired reflective conversations can quickly add up to a lot of reflection from various angles in a short space of time. Your choice of methods will partly depend on how important it is that everyone meets everyone else.

- Milling about (for one-to-one feedback): find a partner; give each other one positive statement about their contribution to the team exercise; find a new partner and repeat, etc.
- Brief encounters (questions and partners keep changing): each person starts with a unique question on a card and finds a partner. Each person answers their partner's question. They swap cards and each finds a new partner.
- Surveys (small groups specialise in one question): subgroups scatter throughout the whole group conducting brief one-to-one interviews on the topic in which they are specialising. Subgroups meet together again to collate the answers and report back their findings to the whole group.
- Mad Hatter's tea party: two lines face each other. People talk with the person standing opposite. At a given signal, everyone moves one to the left and starts talking with their new partner. The facilitator announces a fresh question at each move. If the group is too big to complete a full cycle, set up a suitable number of smaller groups.
- Concentric circles: this is much the same idea as the Mad Hatter's tea party, but is a little easier to set up and manage. This structure does not allow participants to have conversations with people in their own circle, but it does provide an effective way of meeting and learning one-to-one with everyone in another group.
- Matrix meetings: each individual has a list of everyone's names. They place a mark beside the name of anyone they work with on a paired-reviewing exercise of (say) five minutes or more. From time to time they also enter this information on a single-group matrix that builds up a picture of who has worked with whom. A number or letter code can be used to give basic information about who took which role during the exercise (e.g. L=learner, F=facilitator, S= shared). If the target is to complete the matrix, remember to provide enough opportunities for paired reviewing for this to be achievable.

Not all pairings work well – one person can dominate, trust may be low, pairs may decide to take easy options, or just go through the motions or may even opt out. Group facilitators may try to avoid the risks of paired reviews not working well by keeping everyone together under their own watchful eye for whole group reflection. But whole group reflection has its own risks and disadvantages (such as lack of personal space, less personal attention and less airtime for each individual). The challenge is to find the right mix (and sequence) of different group sizes (including reflective time alone) so that there is a good balance between these different 'social settings' for reflection.

ACTIVITY 3.6

Identify the stages and tasks that a student experiences whilst on placement. Highlight how you will integrate reflection throughout each stage and task.

Summary

In summary, reflection is central to the learning experience. This unit has considered what reflection is and how it can be used in the learning process. The barriers to reflection and the role of the facilitator in mentoring the reflective process is also identified and discussed. How we can learn from specific events and the different strategies that may be adopted to assist in the reflective process have also been identified. A number of activities have been presented throughout this unit to assist you in applying the theory to your own situation. The References list should also assist you in obtaining more information about reflection in and on the workplace.

References

Alsop, A. and Ryan, S. (1999) *Making the Most of Fieldwork Education: A Practical Approach*. Stanley Thornes.

Boud, D., Cressey, P. and Docherty, P. (2006) *Productive Reflection at Work*. Taylor & Francis.

Brockbank, A. and McGill, I. (1998) Facilitating Reflective Learning in Higher Education. *Higher Education* 39(4): 489–491.

Brockett, R. G. and Hiemstra, R. (1991) *Self-Direction in Adult Learning: Perspectives on Theory, Research and Practice*. Routledge.

Chimera, K. D. (2007) The Use of Reflective Journals in the Promotion of Reflection and Learning in Post-registration Nursing Students. *Nurse Education Today* 27(3): 192–202.

Dewey, J. (2009) *How We Think*. Biblio Bazaar.

Fade, S. (2012) *Learning and Assessing through Reflection*. http://www.science.ulster.ac.uk/nursing/mentorship/docs/learning/RoyalBromptonV3.pdf.

Gillings, B. (2000) Clinical Supervision in Reflective Practice. Cited in Burns S and Bulman C, *Reflective Practice in Nursing*. Blackwell Science.

Johns, C. (2005) Reflection on the Relationship between Technology and Caring. *Nursing in Critical Care* 10(3): 150–155.

Kemmis, S. (1985) Action Research and the Politics of Reflection. In Boud D, Keough R and Walker D, *Reflection: Turning Experience into Learning*. Kogan Page.

Kolb, D. A. (1984) *Experiential Learning: Experience as the Source of Learning and Development*. Prentice-Hall.

Louden, W. (1991) *Understanding Teaching*. Cassell.

McClure, P. (2012) *Reflection on Practice*. http://www.science.ulster.ac.uk/nursing/mentorship/docs/learning/reflectiononpractice.pdf

Mezirow, J. (1981) A Critical Theory of Adult Learning and Education. *Adult Education* 32(1): 3–24.

Powell, E. (2005) *Reflective Practice*. Taylor & Francis.

Reid, B. (1993) 'But We're Doing it Already'. Exploring a Response to the Concept of Reflective Practice in order To Improve its Facilitation. *Nurse Education Today* 13: 305–309.

Richardson, G. and Maltby, M. (1995) Reflection-on-Practice: Enhancing Student Learning. *Journal of Advanced Nursing* 22(2): 235–242.

Rowntree, D. (1992) *Exploring Open and Distance Learning*. Routledge.

Schon, D. (1987) *Educating the Reflective Practitioner*. Josey Bass.

Assessment in the workplace

Introduction

A key aspect of the work-based facilitator's role is student assessment. Successful supervision requires the facilitator to know why there is a need to assess learning, different approaches to assessment, what is a reliable and valid assessment and how to use feedback to enhance student learning. This unit will identify the skills required to assess in the workplace and assist you in managing students' success and failure.

Aim of the unit

This unit aims to help you understand the nature of assessment in facilitating learning in the workplace.

Outcomes of the unit

At the end of this unit you will be able to:

1   investigate the need for assessment
2   analyse and compare the types of assessment in the workplace
3   redefine assessment and constructive feedback as an aid to learning
4   demonstrate skills essential for effective assessment
5   manage failing students in the workplace
6   plan, implement and evaluate assessment in the workplace.

ACTIVITY 4.1

Throughout this chapter, reflect on three students whom you have assessed: one who is doing very well, one who is meeting the requirements of the placement, and one who is excelling in the workplace. Give a brief description of each student:

- Student One, who is doing very well
- Student Two, who is meeting the requirements of the placement
- Student Three, who is excelling.

(You may wish to include this information and how it has been applied to the unit's materials in your portfolio.)

The need for assessment

Students are assessed for a number of reasons, including motivating students (Oxford Centre for Staff and Learning Development 2011), diagnosing students' strengths and weaknesses, enabling students to identify their strengths and weaknesses (Howard 2006), monitoring student progress (Marsh *et al.* 2010), determining the extent to which students have achieved specific learning objectives, grading student learning, providing a way to judge when a student is competent to practise or proceed on a course (Whittington 2007), informing the nature of feedback to students on their progress, evaluating effectiveness of teaching and planning future teaching to facilitate student progress.

ACTIVITY 4.2

Outline your responsibilities in assessing students' learning in your workplace.

Types of assessment

Two key principles of any assessment are that the assessment is based upon agreed criteria which the student is aware of and that assessment is a continuous process in which a single incident should not 'make or mar' any final judgment.

The assessment process has both a formative and a summative component.

Formative assessment is diagnostic in nature and is concerned with the development of the student, with identifying strengths and weaknesses and with providing the student with feedback on their progress during the learning process. It contains a continuing and systematic appraisal of a student to determine the degree of mastery of a given learning task and to help the student and teacher to focus on the particular learning necessary to achieve mastery. Continuous assessment generally means intermittent assessment, but the focus is on the needs of the individual student, not in terms of pass or fail, but in terms of whether the learning outcome criteria have been met or not. It should also identify the strengths of students' performance and areas that require improvement. The nature of formative assessment is essentially diagnostic (Marsh *et al.* 2010).

Food Forum (2008) believes that it is important that formative assessment

- is embedded in the teaching and learning process of which it is an essential part
- shares learning goals with students
- helps students to understand and recognise the standards to aim for
- provides feedback that helps students to identify what they should do next to improve
- has a commitment that every student can improve
- involves both teacher and students reviewing and reflecting on performance and progress together
- involves students in self-assessment.

Summative assessment is a final assessment that occurs at the end of an experience and is decision-making in nature. It consists of an assessment of the extent to which a student has achieved the outcomes/objectives for a work-based placement as a whole, or a substantial part of it, and contributes to the grading of a student.

ACTIVITY 4.3

What tasks and areas of learning in your workplace do you formatively assess?

What tasks and areas of learning in your workplace do you summatively assess?

Assessment can also be categorised as either a criterion- or norm-referenced type of assessment. In criterion-referenced assessment, particular abilities, skills or behaviours are each specified as a criterion that must be reached. Williams (2009) states that in recent years the focus of interest in work-based learning has moved onto competency standards, sometimes defined as occupational and employment-related standards. This means that placement outcomes are defined in terms of *outcomes* to be achieved by students. In turn, assessment is linked to the criteria expressed in the competency standards. A number of implications flow from this. First, assessment takes on a problem-centred rather than merely a knowledge-based orientation. To prove competency means having to *demonstrate* the attainment of skills and attitudes, not just having to write about them. Secondly, assessment becomes not merely a means of judging knowledge and performance, but an integral part of the learning process itself. Consequently, the emergence of performance-based assessment suggests that we are moving towards assessment that is:

- Standards- or criterion-referenced. Judging outcomes against these pre-defined standards is relatively straightforward.
- Direct and authentic, related directly to the work situation. This has the potential for motivating learning, since learners can see a direct relevance between what is learnt and what is assessed.

The driving test is the classic example of a criterion-referenced test. The examiner has a list of criteria each of which must be satisfactorily demonstrated in order to pass – completing a three-point turn without hitting either kerb, for example. The important thing is that failure in one criterion cannot be compensated for by above-average performance in others; neither can you fail despite meeting every criterion simply because everybody else that day surpassed the criteria and was better than you (Oxford Centre for Staff Learning and Development 2011).

Norm-referenced assessment makes judgments on how well the individual did in relation to others who took the test, and often used in conjunction with this is the curve of 'normal distribution' which assumes that a few will do exceptionally well and a few will do badly and the majority will peak in the middle, normally judged as average. This approach is rarely used in work-based assessment.

A number of specific types of assessment can be used in the assessment of work-based learning. Performance assessment is particularly appropriate for work-based assessment because of features that include:

- students employing higher-order thinking skills (students apply knowledge and skills to solve problems, to synthesise, to explain, etc.)
- depth of knowledge (understanding of a concept, topic, or skill is not superficial)
- connectedness to work (problems/topics are ones that occur in the workplace)
- substantive conversation (teacher–student conversation is two-way and meaningful)
- social support for student achievement, i.e. teachers and peers.

Another example is the use of reviews, which provides an excellent opportunity to refocus all parties on the plans developed at the start of the learning programme and previously agreed targets. If agreed targets have not been met, discussions should focus on developing new action plans and tackling problem areas. Learners benefit from being encouraged to reflect on their progress both on and off the job. Instances have been seen of learners recording their thoughts and achievements in journals that are discussed with their line manager during reviews and used to identify further training and support needs, which learners may find motivating.

These reviews can involve production of a portfolio, which showcases students' growth, experiences, and achievement. It consists of:

- self-selected, representative samples of the student's work
- written justifications for these selections
- formal presentation of the justified selections to peers and teachers.

The primary purpose of a student portfolio is to create an environment where students increasingly reflect upon, assess and control their own growth according to course outcomes and goals. To promote this, the portfolio involves collaboration between teachers and students, with teachers structuring the planning, establishment and implementation of portfolios, and students taking responsibility for the particulars of their own portfolios. Portfolio assessment values the process as well as the products of learning. The unit on Reflection explores the principles underpinning the nature of a portfolio.

Another approach to assessment in the workplace involves the use of a learning contract. Hiemstra (2011) believes that the use of learning contracts enables students to learn on their own initiative, resulting in learning that will be deep and permanent. The process of developing a learning contract involves:

- diagnosis of learning needs
- specification of learning objectives
- identifying learning resources and strategies
- stating target dates for completing activities
- specifying evidence of achievement
- articulating how evidence will be validated
- reviewing the contract with the work-based facilitator
- implementing the contract
- evaluating learning.

Students may find it impossible to produce written evidence for the assessment. The assessor may want to identify other effective ways to overcome this situation, for example, including photographs, videos and CDs as evidence. Mobile device technology gives students greater scope in how they collect evidence.

When to use a particular assessment?

Performance assessment is particularly relevant to work-based learning as it requires students to demonstrate that they have mastered specific skills and competencies by performing or producing something.

The use of a portfolio approach to assessment can assist students to think about their learning whilst on a work-based placement. Furthermore, it can motivate students, provide facilitators with specific examples of a student's learning, help students self-assess their progress and also facilitate self-reflection.

Race (2005) identifies concerns about the assessment process, which can be used to inform decisions about when and how to assess students. These concerns include the belief that assessment is often done in a rush and may be rarely conducted under the best of conditions. Assessment tends to be governed by 'what is easy to assess' and so may omit to provide detailed insight about students' ability. Students rarely know the intimate details of the assessment criteria, and how they will be interpreted. Another concern is, How do we assess unassessable qualities? What competences are measured by assessment anyway? Are they 'can do' competences? Or are they simply 'did do, once' ghosts? What should the assessment be trying to measure?

One way of addressing some of these concerns has been identified by Marsh *et al.* (2010), who believe that there should be formal staging posts in work-based assessment. A minimum expectation would be that this process should involve an initial interview, which includes a student self-assessment, and which should occur at the start of the work-based placement, followed by a mid-placement assessment interview and then a final assessment interview. Lengthy placements of perhaps a year, common in some professions, will obviously require more interim staging posts for assessment.

Many of Race's points need to be considered when undertaking work-based assessment. Another key element of the assessment is the need to tell students how they performed in an assessment. The next part of this unit will explore how this can be done effectively.

ACTIVITY 4.4

You are constantly assessing students' knowledge, skills and attitudes. Consider the following six problems and identify how you would deal with each problem.

Problem 1: professionalism

Another member of staff tells you, 'The other day I saw your student being surly and rude to a patient.'

How would you respond?

Problem 2: time keeping

A colleague complains to you about a student you are supervising: 'You're supposed to be her facilitator. See if you can get her to come back from break on time.'

How would you respond?

Problem 3: dealing with conflict

You hear a colleague 'tearing strips' off your student for some misdemeanour.

How would you respond?

Problem 4: failure to fail

Your third-year student is due a final Practice Assessment. You are concerned about her fitness to practise. On reviewing her progress reports she had previously achieved a satisfactory standard of competence.

What do you do?

Problem 5: poor performance/providing feedback

The student you have been assigned to supervise is causing you concern because he is not showing any initiative or ability to communicate with staff.

How would you deal with this student?

Problem 6: toxic mentorship

You are a facilitator and you observe that a colleague who is also a facilitator seems to have a negative attitude to the students assigned on placement. She is treating them as 'pairs of hands', constantly expecting them to run errands and criticising their ability. You have witnessed her dumping what she calls 'menial' duties on them and blocking their opportunities to be involved in key learning experiences.

What action do you take?

(Adapted from University of Ulster/Queens University Mentorship Training pack)

Possible ways of dealing with these problems can be found at the end of this section.

Giving feedback

Giving feedback is the process of telling another individual how they are perceived (Sharp *et al*. 2010). It can be a source of anxiety for both giver and receiver. The following guidelines for giving useful feedback may help to reduce this anxiety, improve performance, increase morale and help develop teamwork. The risks of poor-quality feedback are that it might demoralise, reduce confidence and even cause conflict.

ACTIVITY 4.5

Can you think from your own experience of one positive experience of getting feedback from a student you supported during their placement?

What contributed to making this a positive experience?

Can you think of a negative experience of getting feedback from a student you supported?

What contributed to making this a negative experience?

Outline anything you would do differently? (You may want to include this in your portfolio.)

Some useful tips, adapted from the work of JISCinfoNET (2012), Sharp *et al.* (2010) and Whittington (2007), for giving students good quality feedback include:

- Ask the student to self-assess first.

- Give praise before criticism.

- Limit what you cover.

- Concentrate on what can be changed.

- Give the student time to think and respond.

- Be clear and specific, not vague.
  Try to be clear about what the feedback is that you want to give. If you are vague then you are likely to increase the anxiety in the receiver and to be misunderstood. The receiver may feel attacked and react defensively. Focus on the assessment criteria.
  Comment on specific behaviours and achievements rather than giving general comments that are hard to learn from. It is not very useful to say to someone, 'You didn't use the flipchart very well.' It's much more useful to say, 'It was difficult to read what you had written on the flipchart because your writing was rather small and the pen you used had a thin tip.'

- Give regular feedback and avoid delay.
  It is useful to receive feedback regularly. Try to give feedback as close to the event as possible. Delay in giving feedback can result in storing up grievances and then delivering them all at once, which can be difficult to cope with. Feedback is only useful if it is given in time for the person to do something about any identified problems. It should focus on something that can be changed.

- Own the feedback you give.
  The feedback you give is your own perception and not an ultimate truth. It is helpful if it is phrased as such: 'I noticed...', 'I find you...', 'I feel...', rather than 'You are...', 'You didn't...'.

- Give balanced constructive feedback.
  Students need to know what they've done right, or well. They need to know this so that they'll keep on doing it right or well, and also because it will make them feel appropriately good about themselves and their work, which in itself aids learning as well as feeling good. They also need to know why it was right or good. Learners sometimes do well by accident, so tell them why it was right or good, in what respects it was right or good. Positive feedback needs to be:

- Clear: don't beat about the bush. If you think it was 'great' or 'excellent' or 'admirable' or 'very stimulating', then say so. Have the courage of your convictions. (Don't worry about using clichés!)
- Specific: words like 'great' or 'excellent' carry a strong emotional message, but when the emotional buzz fades, the intellectual hunger remains. As suggested above, say what, exactly what, was good and say why it was good.
- Personal: that is, make the person you're giving feedback to feel acknowledged as an individual. This will get easier as you get to know your students. Using their name in the feedback helps: 'Emma, I thought the way you handled this was both valid and original. I particularly liked the way you...'.
- Honest: as well as being truthful, honest good news clearly distinguishes between fact and judgement. A numerical answer is 'right'; this is a fact. A design was undertaken 'rigorously'; this is an opinion, although hopefully based on clear criteria for 'rigour'. An argument was 'original'; a fact, at any rate relative to your own current knowledge. An argument was 'elegant'; an opinion, or at any rate a judgement. Be clear what the nature of your good news is.

- Positive feedback improves confidence; it feels good and increases motivation. It may help the receiver to have the confidence to deal with the more negative aspects of their performance.

- Negative feedback, when given in a constructive way, has the greatest impact on changing behaviour and improving performance. Recipients of negative feedback also need to know what they've done wrong, or poorly, or performed in some other way which is inappropriate. And, immediately and always, they need to know in what respects it was wrong or poor or inappropriate, and they need suggestions on ways in which it could have been correct or better.

- Think of the language you are using – use questions initially rather than accusations. For example: 'How do you think reacting like that appeared to the client?', rather than 'That was unprofessional behaviour.'

- Offer support and challenge.
  There are two dimensions to feedback: support and challenge. The most constructive feedback is high on support and high on challenge.

- Explore alternatives.

- Note how the feedback is received.

- Anticipate an emotional response.
  Make time for the feedback and consider when might be a good time to give feedback. Ensure privacy, be supportive but don't get distracted from your aims.

- End on a positive note.
  Round off your feedback with a high note and encouragement. 'You really seem to be getting to grips with this'; 'Your analytic skills are improving steadily'; 'You're making good use of evidence'. Say whatever you can that's encouraging and truthful.

The majority of feedback that is given is verbal. However, there will be times when you are required to give written feedback. This may be when you are giving a student feedback on their performance as part of a formal or final (summative) assessment of the student's performance or as evidence in their assessment documentation. The previous guidance still applies. It is helpful if written feedback is specific, constructive and owned. It is also most helpful if it is given regularly rather than only at the end of a placement when the student has little opportunity to respond to it.

Feedback may need to be about specific achievements or generally regarding the student's qualities. Try and write your feedback to the student rather than about them and ensure you use 'judgement' and evaluative words rather than just stating what the student has done or what they have achieved. It is important to get across 'how well' they performed.

Examples of good feedback from Sharp *et al.* (2010) are:

'Jose, as we have discussed you show clear initiative in setting your goals. You have in the main approached the (specifics) activities with a professional and considered approach.'

'The feedback from the clients demonstrated that you had excellent communication skills and were able to pick up on non-verbal as well as verbal cues in a supportive and helpful manner. We discussed the need for your documentation of client issues to be more specific and although you have responded to feedback there is still scope for it to be more detailed.'

'My observations of you in practice showed that you have a meticulous approach to detail and that you are able to prioritise well.'

Giving effective feedback is a key part of the assessment process, but it is important to recognise that this is not the only skill that a work-based facilitator needs to ensure good quality assessment. The next section will examine some of the other skills that are fundamental to assessment.

ACTIVITY 4.6

Plan a feedback session for your previously identified three students using the above information. It would be useful to note points in their performance that you would highlight and provide feedback on.

Student One

Student Two

Student Three

(You may want to include this in your portfolio.)

Skills for effective assessment

Work-based facilitators need to identify evidence that represents student competence so that appropriate judgements of student performance are made. In addition, the work-based facilitator may need to document the outcome of such judgements and the basis upon which they have been made. Examine the student assessment documentation for the placement to find out the criteria for assessment and any additional requirements and deadlines:

- Is the assessment continuous/one off?
- What is the expected level of assessment, e.g. formative or summative?

Ensure that you understand the criteria used for assessment and familiarise yourself with the paperwork. Discuss/clarify any concerns you have with university staff or peers/managers. Discuss with the student their understanding, expectations and responsibilities and make explicit what preparation is expected by the student.

Often such judgements are made on the basis of an observation of a student's performance. This may then be followed by a process of questioning the student, a skill that has been previously covered in the Supporting learning in the workplace unit. Sharp *et al.* (2010) identify a number of facets of effective observation in the workplace:

- Prepare and then ensure the student knows what you are observing and when and how you will give feedback. Before an observation it is useful for the two people involved to meet for around 20 minutes to discuss the objectives/intended student learning for the session.
- Think about the impact of your presence during the activity and discuss it with the student; consider nervousness, location, practicality. As an observer, you need to try to sit in an unobtrusive position, but where you can see and record the student behaviour.
- If it is relevant, then consider informing the clients/others that you will be observing the student so that they understand the facilitator and student roles. Clarify with the student when you may intervene (i.e. client safety). Ask the student to describe what the activity was and then ask them to evaluate it (use reflective frameworks if you wish).
- The facilitator should review his/her notes as soon as possible after the observation before discussing the activity with the student. The feedback should be specific and prompt. Describe your observations:
  - Say what you saw – the facts.
  - Describe your interpretation of your observations and link this to the assessment criteria (Oxford Centre for Staff Learning and Development 2011).
  - Say what you think.
  - These are your judgements and impressions (based on your knowledge and experience).

One possible outcome of a student assessment, whether formative or summative, could be that the student is not achieving a satisfactory standard. The next part of this unit will consider how a work-based facilitator can help such failing students.

Helping a failing student

ACTIVITY 4.7

What are the signs that would indicate to you that a student may fail their placement?

Why do you think students fail work-based placements?

Duffy (2007a) examined the reasons why nursing students failed on work-based placements. She identified a number of reasons, including:

- Poor communication and interpersonal skills.
- Lack of interest and failure to participate in practice learning.
- Persistent lateness.
- Lack of personal insight.
- Lack of insight into professional boundaries.

Marsh *et al.* (2010) believe that failing a student is difficult for a number of reasons. For example:

- There are emotional issues involved.
- Supporting a failing student is time-consuming.
- You may feel responsible for the failing student.
- You may want to take the student's personal circumstances into account (this may or may not be appropriate).
- Inexperienced assessors lack confidence in failing a student.

The consequences are that students are successfully passing a work-based placement when there is doubt about their ability. There are some students who reach the end of their course and then fail (which has a more devastating effect). Clients may be put at risk from unsafe practitioners.

Therefore, a student should fail when that student has been given detailed and regular feedback on areas of poor performance and has been made aware of the areas of concern and how to improve performance, but does not respond or act on feedback regarding their performance; or when the student fails to provide evidence of meeting the required standard (when the opportunity is available); or when the student acts in an unprofessional or unsafe way despite feedback and support.

ACTIVITY 4.8
What action do you take to support students who are struggling?

There are a number of strategies that can be used to help support the student who appears to be failing. Marsh et *al.* (2010) and Sharp *et al.* (2010) identify a range of methods that a work-based facilitator could use:

- early exploration and intervention with the student, e.g. ask why they appear to lack interest or are constantly late
- avoiding making assumptions and jumping to conclusions
- clear articulation of expectations
- prompt removal of obstacles to allow facilitation of progress
- negotiation of learning opportunities
- not being afraid of your 'gut feelings': respond to the cues you have
- not giving the benefit of the doubt! Acknowledge the 'alarm bells'!
- asking colleagues for their views (especially those with more experience)
- seeking support and advice early from university staff and clinical managers or experienced assessors
- adopting an approach of giving consistent and regular positive and constructive negative feedback
- asking the student to self-assess – ask them to say how they think they are performing (in relation to specific areas or generally)
- getting help in articulating the problems (particularly with unsatisfactory student attitude)
- being clear about what you think the issue or problem is and trying to give examples
- relating the examples to behaviours and observations rather than impressions or reports from others
- documenting problems/issues early
- developing a plan of action with specific objectives to support the student (specifying responsibilities of all involved)
- Discussing with others and seeking support in dealing with students/your own emotional responses
- Recognising your accountability and responsibility to fail a student (Duffy 2007b).

However, these strategies may not always be successful. If this happens, then according to Marsh *et al.* (2010), a work-based facilitator needs to:

- give formal written feedback at an early stage
- arrange a tripartite meeting with the student and appropriate parties from the student's higher education institution
- develop an action plan agreed by all parties
- arrange regular formal meetings with the student(s) to discuss progress during the placement
- give the student every opportunity and support to progress
- recognise that some students need to fail.

Heathfield (2012) and Marsh *et al.* (2010) provide some tips on how to avoid intimidating the student so that the issues can be effectively resolved.

- Create an environment that is conducive to successful conflict resolution. Quiet, private settings work best. Agree prior to sitting down together that the purpose of the meeting is to resolve the conflict. When you make this agreement, all parties arrive prepared.
- If you feel it will be a difficult situation and would like moral support, then arrange for a colleague who knows and has worked with the student to join you. Make sure the student knows who is going to be there in advance of the meeting. They might feel quite threatened if you go in 'mob-handed' without their prior knowledge.
- Ensure all the required assessment documentation is completed accurately and that all your previous meetings and the outcomes of those meetings are recorded as fully as possible.
- From the outset, try to create a safe and friendly environment by being relaxed and as informal as possible. Do not, of course, overdo this as you are ultimately going to give the student bad news and it would be rather cruel to lull them into a false sense of security.
- Determine what outcomes you'd like to see as a result of the discussion. A better working relationship? A better solution to the problem? A broadened understanding of each person's needs and wants? Thoughtful solutions and outcomes are infinite if you are creative.
- Begin by allowing each party to express their point of view. A useful opening strategy is to turn the focus onto the student by asking them their views on their progress. If they are aware of the problems during the practice placement, ask the student to carry out a self-assessment either on paper or verbally. You may save yourself considerable time and anxiety if the student is self-aware enough to tell you why they may not have performed their best and identifies for you where the student thinks the areas of weaknesses are. If the student is lacking in self-awareness then this strategy has limited value, but it does allow the student to have a voice before you break the bad news.
- The purpose of the exchange is to make sure both parties clearly understand the viewpoint of the other. Make sure each party ties their opinions to real performance data and other facts, where possible. This is not the time to discuss; it is the time to ask questions, clarify points for better understanding and truly hear the student's viewpoint.
- As previously stated, it is quite constructive in giving feedback to someone who has not performed well to provide feedback in what is sometimes called a 'praise sandwich'. Start by giving the student something positive about their progress and performance; then discuss areas that need improvement. Complete your feedback with another positive statement.
- Allow the student to question what you have said and discuss any issues they may have until they feel they understand the outcome.
- Agree on the difference in the points of view. You must agree on the problem together to begin to search for a solution. Often problems are simply misunderstandings. Try to focus on the issues, not the personalities of the participants. Don't 'you' each other as in, 'You always...'.
- Explore and discuss potential solutions and alternatives. Try to focus on both your individual needs and wants and the student. After all, if one person 'wins', that means the other person 'loses'. Students who feel as if they have lost are not effective learners, but will harbour resentment and may even sabotage the relationship. Make sure you discuss the positive and negative possibilities of each suggestion, before you reject any suggested solutions.
- Agree on a plan that meets the needs of all parties. Agree on follow-up steps, as necessary, to make the plan work. Agree on what each person will do to resolve the situation. Set clear goals and know how you will measure success. Provide the student with advice on how they could improve future performance.
- Complete necessary documentation.
- Do what you agreed to do.

If a student fails to improve and reach a satisfactory standard, then it is important that the work-based facilitator informs the relevant member(s) of staff in the student's higher education institution so that appropriate action concerning the student's progress on the course can be taken.

ACTIVITY 4.9

Review your own performance as an assessor, using the Communication Skills Questionnaire in the Appendix at the end of this unit.

Identify your strengths and areas that require further development.

What action will you take to further develop your assessment skills? (You may want to include this in your portfolio.)

Evaluating an assessment

An important consideration in assessing work-based learning is to examine how useful an assessment has been. North Central Regional Educational Laboratory (2010) argues that a work-based assessment should avoid tasks that may be merely interesting activities for students, but may not yield evidence of a student's mastery of the desired outcomes. It is important to match assessment tasks to intended learning outcomes so that assessment matches specific instructional intentions, adequately represents the skills that students should attain and enables students to demonstrate their progress and capabilities.

Furthermore, the assessment should measure achievement of all learning outcomes, enable a student to demonstrate excellence, not discriminate against individual students (a topic that is explored in detail within the Diversity unit) and be able to be generalised to predict student performance in other situations. One way of avoiding discrimination is to use a diverse range of assessment instruments and processes, so as not to disadvantage any particular individual or group of learners (Fowell *et al.* 1999).

There are a number of key concepts underpinning any evaluation of the assessment process.

Validity

JISCinfoNET (2012) describes this as the degree to which you are able to measure what you think you are measuring. Atherton (2011) believes that assessment methods should be chosen so that they directly measure that which it is intended to measure, and not just a reflection of the knowledge, skills or competences being assessed.

Three dimensions of validity are construct validity, content validity and predictive validity.

Construct validity is concerned with the measurement of abstract concepts and traits, such as ability, anxiety, attitude, knowledge, etc. Given that one of the objectives of work-based learning is to encourage the development of the reflective practitioner, then the abstract notion of 'reflection' could, in principle, also be measured and assessed. Before any trait can be measured, however, it has to be operationally defined. Taking each trait, the programme developer proceeds to elaborate on all of the characteristics that make up that trait. For example, using our example of reflection, this could be characterised as the ability to recognise one's own strengths and weaknesses, to value one's own positive achievements and to produce plans for new action and self-development based on previous reflection.

Content validity is an estimate of the extent to which an assessment tool takes items from the subject domain being addressed, including not only cognitive topics but also behaviours. For this to be achievable, it is necessary to define accurately the content domain and its boundaries. So, for example, producing a test on how to use the drawing facility in Microsoft Word might be relatively straightforward, since this is a routine procedure. But taking a work-based learning topic such as 'project management' might not be so simple, as it is a broad and complex subject. Is there such a thing as project management in the abstract, or are the subjects of project management in engineering and project management as a management tool for business planning quite distinct? The principles and practice of project management may be quite different according to the operational context.

Predictive validity shows how well a test can forecast future job performance or attainment. There is little point in a test having both construct and content validity if it fails to identify students who are likely to be 'high performers' in a key work role. It could be argued that predictive validity is of particular importance to organisations that are sponsoring their staff through work-based learning programmes. For most organisations, and particularly those operating in a commercial environment, the financial 'bottom line' is paramount. Like any other activity, sponsorship of a work-based learning programme is seen as a means by which the skills and aptitudes of staff can be developed for the commercial benefit of the organisation. It is important, then, when work-based learning assessment processes identify someone as a 'high performer', that this is translated into high performance activity in the workplace.

In practical terms, work-based facilitators get as close as possible to the student's actual performance and also ensure that any evidence that a student produces is recent and that it belongs to that student. Often students need to transfer work-based learning from one context to another. The Oxford Centre for Staff Learning Development (2011) believes this is more likely to happen when the contexts are similar and that, to facilitate successful transfer, the activity should have a real purpose and fully represent the reality of the workplace.

Reliability

This refers to the degree to which the rating of student performance on an assessment is consistent over repeated applications of the assessment and therefore free of measurement error. The rating of student performance should be independent of the assessor.

The assessment should have stability, i.e. scores achieved on the same test or assessment instrument taken on two different occasions should be the same or similar. The problem here for work-based learning is that it is difficult to ensure that the same aspects of the same task can be assessed on different occasions in the workplace. Indeed, since one of the objectives of work-based learning is to develop competence during placements, it is change rather than consistency that is required.

There needs to be inter-judge reliability, which compares the consistency of observations when more than one person is judging. An example would be where two assessors judge the quality of a work-based project. The reliability of the observation is provided by the degree to which the views (scores) of each judge correlate. Work-based learning, when involving the judging of competencies, usually requires the collective opinions of both higher education institution staff and work-based facilitators (usually experienced professionals).

Finally there should be intra-judge reliability. This is the extent to which an assessor is consistent when judging across a range of people – for example, assessing several students on a work-based placement. For a competency-based assessment system, a variety of assessment methods need to be used if reliability is to be addressed. These could include a mixture of tasks, projects, presentations, etc.

A practical way to evaluate the reliability of an assessment is to obtain evidence that may have been used in judging a student's performance. One question concerns how much evidence a student needs to produce to demonstrate achievement of stated outcome or competence. There is no easy answer to this question, as the nature of the evidence that the student provides to demonstrate achievement of specific outcomes and competence statements will be very dependent on the nature of the work-based activity. Therefore, the broader the type of evidence, and the context and the number of occasions on which the students produce this evidence, the more likely it will be that the students are able to demonstrate that they have required the level of competence and so increase the reliability of the evidence.

The Oxford Centre for Staff Learning Development (2011) recognises that, whilst complete objectivity is impossible to achieve, it is a goal worth aiming for. To this end, what has been described as the 'connoisseur' approach to assessment (like a wine-taster or tea-blender of many years experience, not able to describe exactly what they are looking for, but 'knowing it when they find it') is no longer acceptable. Explicitness in terms of learning outcomes and assessment criteria is vitally important in attempting to achieve reliability. They should be explicit to both assessor and students when an assessment task is set.

Student problems

You were asked to consider how you would deal with six student problems earlier in this unit. Here are some suggestions about how you might do this, though remember that these are only suggestions and in reality you may find that alternative approaches are more effective.

Problem 1: professionalism

Another member of staff tells you 'The other day I saw your student being surly and rude to a patient.'
How would you respond?

Answer:
Find out from your colleague exactly what she saw and heard.
Ask the student about the alleged incident. The patient confirms that the student was rude.
Take the student to a private area.
Tell the student about the report that has been made.
Ask the student for her/his account of the events. (It may be necessary to have the witness to the behaviour and the lecturer present).
Advise student of the expectation to behave in a professional manner.
Ask the student to be willing to apologise to the patient, accompanied by you as the student's facilitator.
Advise the lecturer of the incident and make a written comment in the student's progress notes or cause-for-concern section.
Arrange regular review of progress to provide feedback.
How this problem is handled will largely depend on the student's response to being confronted about the incident.

Problem 2: time keeping

A colleague complains to you about a student you are supervising: 'You're supposed to be her facilitator. See if you can get her to come back from break on time.'
How would you respond?

Answer:
Take the student to a quiet area.
Find out why the student is consistently late back from breaks.
Ask the student to explain why you are concerned about her lateness on returning from breaks.
Discuss the importance of professional responsibility, reliability and dependability as a member of the team.
Advise the student that you will be monitoring her over a specified period.
Monitor over the next few days.
Advise the relevant university lecturer.
Record the problem in the student's progress notes.

Problem 3: dealing with conflict

You hear a colleague 'tearing strips' off your student for some misdemeanour.
How would you respond?

Answer:

Take the student aside and provide support by asking what happened and listening to the student's concerns.

When the student has calmed down allocate her to work in an area away from the member of staff concerned.

Ensure the student is able to work with someone who will provide professional support.

Ask your colleague to explain why she behaved as she did with the student.

Monitor the student's performance and response.

Explain that, even if the student was in the wrong, you would rather that the criticism was given in a constructive way and, if necessary, through you.

Record the incident and the action taken in the student's progress notes.

Again, how this is handled will depend on how your colleague normally deals with students. Is this 'a one-off' or the way she/he treats everyone (perhaps there is a conflict of personality).

Problem 4: failure to fail

Your third-year student is due a final Practice Assessment. You are concerned about her fitness to practise. On reviewing her progress reports she had previously achieved a satisfactory standard of competence.

What do you do?

Answer:

Discuss with the student her progress in relation to achievement of practice outcomes.

Outline your concerns about the student's performance.

Make contact with the relevant university lecturer to discuss the student's failure to progress.

Arrange a tripartite meeting with the student and lecturer to identify the remedial action required.

Ensure that the student understands what is expected. Record the action required and the timescale for completion.

Agree how the student is to be monitored and when feedback is to be given.

Do this frequently.

Continue to liaise with the lecturer about the student's progress and for support and guidance.

Maintain a record of feedback and the student's response.

Do not be afraid to have the courage of your conventions if you feel the student is not making the grade.

Problem 5: poor performance/providing feedback

The student you have been assigned to supervise is causing you concern because he is not showing any initiative or ability to communicate with staff.

How would you deal with this student?

Answer:

Discuss with the student his progress in relation to achievement of practice outcomes.

Ask the student to assess his own performance to date.

Outline your concerns about the student's performance and in particular the failure to show any initiative or communicate with staff or patients.

Find out if there are any mitigating circumstances, e.g. difficulties in the student's personal circumstances that are particularly difficult to deal with.

Make contact with the relevant university lecturer to discuss the student's failure to progress.

Arrange a tripartite meeting and identify the remedial action required and the support that will be given.

Ensure that the student understands what is expected. Record the action required and the timescale for completion.

Agree how the student is to be monitored and when feedback is to be given.

Do this frequently.

Continue to liaise with the lecturer about the student's progress and for support and guidance. Maintain a record of feedback and the student's response.

Do not be afraid to have the courage of your convictions if you feel that the student is not making the grade.

Problem 6: toxic mentorship

You are a facilitator and you observe that a colleague who is also a facilitator seems to have a negative attitude to the students assigned on placement. She is treating them as 'pairs of hands', constantly expecting them to run errands and criticising their ability. You have witnessed her dumping what she calls 'menial' duties on them and blocking their opportunities to be involved in key learning experiences.

What action do you take?

Answer:

Report this to the relevant manager as the facilitator has a duty to facilitate students to develop competence in practice.

The offending facilitator will need to be spoken to and given the opportunity to explain why she/he had such a negative attitude.

Examine the relationship between the facilitator and students.

Perhaps the facilitator feels threatened and needs support and/or updating.

It may be necessary not to allocate students to this person for a period.

Assign the students to another facilitator to ensure a supportive learning experience?

Additional training in supervising students may be necessary for this facilitator.

Conclusion

This section has examined various aspects of assessment in the workplace. One feature of the assessment process is the use of reflection, e.g. students reflect upon their progress in relation to informal and formal assessment activity, and facilitators observe students and reflect upon the adequacy of student performance and consider where improvement is required. The previous unit examines the nature of reflection in the workplace in more detail, the next unit looks at how students develop ability to work with others in the workplace.

Appendix

Complete the communication questionnaire (Department of Health 2005) in Table 4.1. Score your responses on the response sheet (Table 4.2). Transfer your 'Yes' and 'No' answers for each of the 48 statements to the relevant boxes. Add up the number of 'Yes' answers for each column and write the total in the blank box at the bottom of each column.

Each score will represent how you conform to the particular style of communication (see Table 4.3). If you score six or more 'Yes' answers for a category, then this suggests that you have a natural tendency to use this style.

- Consider the descriptions.
- Consider the implications.
- Consider the implications for your *own development* and facilitation style.
- Consider how:
  - others may see you
  - your style may cause tension for others
  - you can use your strengths
  - to avoid the traps your style may cause.
- Look at the other descriptions and consider how you can:
  - make others more comfortable
  - observe and learn how others respond to you
  - make changes to improve communications with individuals who you have the most 'difficulty' with.

Table 4.1 Communication questionnaire

	Start here	Yes/no
01	Do you think it is a sign of strength not to show emotions during a crisis?	
02	Do you often interrupt people when you think they are incorrect?	
03	Does it annoy you when people try to cheer you up?	
04	If you ask someone to do something and they do it wrong, do you have a go at them?	
05	When others have little to say are you able to keep a conversation going?	
06	Are you proud of your ability to deal with people?	
07	Do tactful people annoy you because you wish people would say exactly what they mean?	
08	When you are down in the dumps, do lively people make you feel even worse?	
09	Do you try to sound confident even when you are unsure about the facts?	
10	Are you impatient with people who like to discuss their motives?	
11	Do you think that your feelings are too deep to discuss with others?	
12	Do you keep quiet when you feel you may offend someone?	
13	Are you diplomatic when you have to tell others to do something against their will?	
14	Does it bother you when others correct your mistakes?	
15	Do you find it difficult to discuss your problems with others?	
16	Are you embarrassed by people who talk about their feelings?	
17	Do you believe people when they ask you if you are all right?	
18	Do you find it hard to admit to your mistakes?	
19	Do you believe that people take advantage of those who are considerate?	
20	Do you value good manners in others?	
21	Do you feel immediately inclined to tell others when something exciting happens to you?	
22	Do you hate to be taken for a ride?	
23	Do you pride yourself on your ability to put up with setbacks?	
24	If someone asked you not to disturb them would you feel hurt?	
25	Are you often first to speak when an opinion is requested?	
26	Do you enjoy being provocative?	
27	Do you think that being blunt is harmful?	
28	Do you get bored with conversations that don't concern you?	
29	Do you feel that people don't understand you?	
30	Do you like to be the centre of attention?	
31	Do you treat conversations as a chance to test your mettle against others?	
32	If a colleague has a different opinion from yours, will you try to win them over to your point of view?	
33	Do you think that people should keep their problems to themselves?	
34	Do you find it hard to keep a secret?	
35	Do you ignore people when they make you angry?	
36	If a colleague is unhappy would you actively discuss their problems?	
37	If you have a problem, would you silently worry about it, even during an evening out?	
38	Does it annoy you to hear someone else dominating a conversation?	
39	Do you worry about whether other people like you?	
40	Do you resent being asked what you are thinking or feeling?	
41	Do you think that your colleagues ought to know what makes you tick?	
42	Do you visibly show your emotions?	
43	Would you hate to show your distress in front of a colleague?	
44	When you have some time alone, do you spend much of it on the telephone?	
45	Do you find advice from others irritating?	
46	Will you say almost anything to fill a lull in a conversation?	
47	Do you see it as your responsibility to keep other people happy?	
48	Do you often find other people oversensitive?	

Source: Department of Health (2005)

Table 4.2 Communication questionnaire score sheet

Response sheet

04	02	03	05	01	06
07	09	08	21	10	12
17	14	11	24	16	13
19	18	15	28	23	20
22	25	29	30	33	27
26	32	35	34	36	39
31	38	37	44	40	41
48	45	42	46	43	47
Aggressive	Dominating	Worrying	Talkative	Quietly confident	Hinting

Source: Department of Health (2005)

Table 4.3 Communication styles

Style	Positives	Negatives
Aggressive	Doesn't get pushed around Clear Focused Results orientated	Uses conversations as a duel to be won Can be argumentative (and likes it) Tries to gain dominance
Dominating	Has a view on everything Usually 'expert' in one area Can step in and take charge Always joins in	Can 'put down' less able people Takes over conversations Not always inclusive of quieter members
Worrying	Always makes allowances Highly emotional Risk analyser	Can be negative Appears withdrawn when thinking Needs time to make decision Emotionally draining
Talkative	Easy to get on with Lots of friends Sociable Non-threatening Sense of humour	Talks too much about nothing Lots of friends Uncomfortable with short silences Talks over quieter members of the group
Quietly confident	Seen as emotionally stable Tower of strength Used as sounding board Confidential	Can be seen as aloof Takes too much on Risk of burnout Can be too self-critical
Hinting	Influences from behind Quiet and thoughtful Gets on with most people	Avoids conflict Doesn't say what they truly mean Can be seen as manipulative by more direct communicators

Source: Department of Health (2005)

References

Atherton, J. S. (2011) *Teaching and Learning; Assessment.* www.learningandteaching.info/teaching/assessment.htm

Duffy, K. (2007a) Supporting Failing Students in Practice 1: Assessment. *Nursing Times* 103(47): 20–12.

Duffy, K. (2007b) Supporting Failing Students in Practice 2: Management. *Nursing Times* 103(48): 28–29.

Food Forum (2008) *Assessment for Learning.* www.foodforum.org.uk/curriculum/Assessment.shtml.

Fowell, S. L., Southgate, L. J. and Bligh, J. (1999) Evaluating Assessment: The Missing Link? *Medical Education.* 33 (4): 276–281.

Heathfield, S. M. (2012) *Why People Avoid Conflict Resolution.* http://humanresources.about.com/cs/conflictresolves/a/conflictcourage.htm

Hiemstra, R. (2011) *Learning Contracts.* www-distance.syr.edu/contract.html

JISCinfoNET (2012) *Characteristics of a 'Good' Assessment Programme.* www.jiscinfonet.ac.uk/InfoKits/effective-use-of-VLEs/e-assessment/assess-characteristics/view

Marsh, S., Cooper, K., Jordan, G., Merrett, S., Scammell, J. and Clark, V. (2010) *Managing Failing Students in Practice.* www.science.ulster.ac.uk/nursing/mentorship/learning_materials.php

North Central Regional Educational Laboratory (2010) *Select or Design Assessments that Elicit Established Outcomes.* www.ncrel.org/sdrs/areas/issues/methods/assment/as7sele2.htm

Oxford Centre for Staff and Learning Development (2011) *Purpose and Principles of Assessment.* www.brookes.ac.uk/services/ocsld/resources/assessment/pandp.html

Race, P. (2005) *Quality of Assessment.* www.londonmet.ac.uk/deliberations/seda-publications/race.cfm.

Sharp, P., Ainslie, T., Hamphill, A., Hobson, S., Merriman, C., Ong, P. and Roche, J. (2010) *Mentoring.* www.science.ulster.ac.uk/nursing/mentorship/learning_materials.php

Whittington C (2007) *Assessment in Social Work: A Guide for Learning and Teaching.* www.scie.org.uk/publications/guides/guide18.

Williams, A. (2009) *Work-based Assessment: A Handbook for University Tutors.* www.heacademy.ac.uk/resources/detail/LLN/GMSA_Work_based_assessment_handbook_for_university_tutors

Working with others in the workplace

Introduction

An important aspect of the world of work is the ability to work with others. This unit is designed to assist you in reflecting upon your skills of working in groups and with others and also in recognising the competencies and skills required by the learner and in developing and enhancing them. A number of terms are used to describe the ways in which people from different disciplines and/or professions learn with each other; these include multi-disciplinary learning, inter-disciplinary learning, shared learning, common learning, multi-professional education and inter-professional education. For the purposes of this unit, the term working with others in the workplace is used to encompass all of these.

Aim of the unit

This unit aims to help you understand the importance of others in the workplace and how they can contribute to student learning.

Outcomes of the unit

At the end of the unit you will be able to:

1 recognise and understand the role of others and their contribution to learning in the workplace
2 discuss the role of groups and individuals in enhancing learning and work in the workplace
3 develop a strategy of dealing with barriers to working with others and how to obtain their cooperation
4 formulate and deliver effective methods of involving others to aid learning in the workplace.

The importance of working with others

Wherever people work together, groups will be formed. People will belong to one or more group, with each group having a different goal and purpose. These groups may be formal or informal. Formal groups are created to complete defined tasks, whilst informal groups are created voluntarily and are made up of individuals with common interests or roles. Informal groups are not usually recognised by the organisation, but they can have a significant impact upon the work of others and can, therefore, be a useful resource when considering learning opportunities for a student.

The work-based facilitator and the student constitute a group and their interaction can reflect the advantages and problems often associated with group interaction.

Four aspects of groups are important to how they function, namely group size, roles of members, group norms and group cohesion.

- Group size: the number of people in a group can affect the dynamic of the group and its effectiveness. Group members are usually more satisfied in small groups, but group performance will depend on the task to be performed.
- Members' roles: various important group roles have been identified by Porteous (2012), including:
  1 Task roles: helping a group to reach its goals.
  2 Maintenance roles: supporting and nurturing other group members.
  3 Self-centred roles: providing self-gratification to individual members even at the expense of the group.
- Group norms: this is the standard of conduct that the group members accept and the rules for what must or must not be done.
- Group cohesion: the member's attraction and loyalty to the group.

ACTIVITY 5.1

Working in groups is an important part of work-based learning. The following activities are designed to help you reflect upon your experiences and how you can help groups work effectively.

As a work-based facilitator, how can you help the student recognise the different groups functioning in the workplace and their roles and responsibilities?

Can you think of a positive experience of working in a group?

What contributed to this being a positive experience?

Can you think of a negative experience of working in a group?

What contributed to this being a negative experience?

How would you summarise your thoughts on how to ensure that groups work effectively?

Roles and responsibilities of individuals and groups

As discussed above, groups come together for many different reasons and in many different ways but, to ensure that individuals can work effectively in the workplace, it is important that they recognise and understand the roles and responsibilities of others and how they contribute to how things can be done efficiently and effectively. Where patients/clients are central to the work it becomes even more important that there are good working relationships, shared outcomes and a planned approach to the service. This can only be achieved by recognising and drawing from the expertise and competencies of all involved whilst not forgetting that the patient/client and families are the most important individuals within this process.

CAIPE (2012) uses the term, 'inter-professional education' (IPE) to include all such learning in academic and work-based settings before and after qualification, adopting an inclusive view of who is a 'professional'. Inter-professional education occurs when two or more professions learn with, from and about each other to improve collaboration and the quality of care.

To assist in identifying which groups and individuals are central to your and the learner's daily work, complete the following activity. Aspects of this activity could also be used with the learner to introduce them to the working team.

ACTIVITY 5.2

Identify the individuals that you interact with in your daily work.

1   Cluster them into their working groups, remembering that most individuals belong to one or more groups.
2   Briefly outline the individuals' roles and responsibilities.
3   Distinguish which of these individuals or groups could contribute to the learning experience.
4   Design an activity to assist the learner in being able to identify the roles and responsibilities of individuals and groups in the workplace and their importance to their learning experience.
5   Evaluate and reflect upon the effectiveness of your plan and make recommendations for its development.

Now that you have identified the individuals you work with and those who can contribute to the learning experience, it is important to have some understanding of the theory of the way in which groups work and come together.

Groups and individuals

Tuckman (1965) identified four stages of group development, adding a fifth stage ten years later.

Stage 1: Forming

In the *Forming* stage, personal relations are characterised by dependence. Group members rely on safe, patterned behaviour and look to the group leader for guidance and direction. Group members have a desire for acceptance by the group and a need to know that the group is safe. Serious topics and feelings are avoided.

To grow from this stage to the next, each member must relinquish the comfort of non-threatening topics and risk the possibility of conflict.

Stage 2: Storming

The next stage, *Storming*, is characterised by competition and conflict in the personal-relations dimension and organisation in the task-functions dimension. As the group members attempt to organise for the task, conflict inevitably affects personal relations. Individuals have to bend and mould their feelings, ideas, attitudes and beliefs to suit the group organisation, often reflecting conflicts over leadership, structure, power and authority.

To progress to the next stage, group members must move to a problem-solving mentality. The most important trait in helping groups to move on to the next stage seems to be the ability to listen.

Stage 3: Norming

In the *Norming* stage, interpersonal relations are characterised by cohesion. Group members are engaged in active acknowledgment of all members' contributions, community-building and maintenance, and solving of group issues. It is during this stage of development (assuming the group gets this far) that people begin to experience a sense of group belonging and a feeling of relief as a result of resolving interpersonal conflicts.

The major task function of stage three is the data flow between group members: They share feelings and ideas, solicit and give feedback to one another and explore actions related to the task. The major drawback of the norming stage is that members may begin to fear the inevitable future breakup of the group; they may resist change of any sort.

Stage 4: Performing

The *Performing* stage is not reached by all groups. If group members are able to evolve to stage four, their capacity, range and depth of personal relations expand to true interdependence. In this stage, people can work independently, in subgroups, or as a total unit with equal facility. There is support for experimentation in solving problems and an emphasis on achievement. The overall goal is productivity through problem-solving and work.

Stage 5: Adjourning

Tuckman's final stage, *Adjourning*, involves the termination of task behaviours and disengagement from relationships. A planned conclusion usually includes recognition for participation and achievement and an opportunity for members to say personal goodbyes.

Tuckman's original work simply described the way he had observed groups, whether they were conscious of it or not. Later work (Tuckman and Jensen 1977) acknowledged that the real value is in recognising where a group is in the process, and helping it to move to the Performing stage. In the real world, groups are often forming and changing and, each time that happens, they can move to a different stage. A group might be happily Norming or Performing, but a new member might force them back into Storming. Leaders will be ready for this, and will help the group get back to Performing as quickly as possible.

Individuals' needs and difference

It is often assumed that we naturally develop the skills to work with others. Good teaching involves working in groups. This does not mean that the individuals within them are working as a team, but implies that learners must be encouraged and given the opportunity to learn these skills.

The aim of the unit is to encourage work-based facilitators to develop and demonstrate their ability to work cooperatively with others to achieve shared objectives. This sharing of objectives is important.

Experience shows that team working:

- increases energy and creativity
- makes the most of a range of skills and knowledge
- improves understanding, communication and a sense of shared purpose
- improves efficiency.

ACTIVITY 5.3

Working in a team requires you to develop a range of communication skills. This activity asks you to engage in an activity and evaluate your role in the group.

Take part in a one-to-one discussion and a group discussion.

Respond appropriately to others.

Adapt what you say to suit different situations.

Listen carefully to what others say.

Develop points and ideas, with an awareness of others' feelings, beliefs and opinions.

Encourage others to contribute.

Listen and respond sensitively.

Respond perceptively to contributions from others.

Evaluate how effective you were in the group and the roles you adopted.

How might you teach these skills to your student?

The main learning experience for students on placement will be that of meeting and working with a completely new group of people, often older than the student and with more authority. While students on work experience may not always have the opportunity to plan their work and develop process skills to any great extent, they should be able to demonstrate their personal qualities and practise and improve their interpersonal skills.

Personal development

The Key Skills Foundation (2005) believes that:

- Working with others is an opportunity for students to demonstrate personal qualities, which are not always fully celebrated in their other areas of study.
- Working with others can be used to support students in tackling issues to do with social, cultural and personal identity, and associated values.
- When students have a framework of skills that makes them more aware of the cooperative skills that they have, they will more likely be aware of the skills they need to develop further.
- The rules and conventions of all social activities require people to cooperate, even when they are competing against each other, as in many kinds of sport. People need to cooperate with each other whether they are planning simply to meet another person or are planning a large-scale social event. While the skills and qualities needed for a successful social life are seldom expressed in the formal terms of working with others, they are nevertheless the same.
- The skill of working with others is intrinsic to our everyday lives and this is reflected in the skills, qualities and knowledge needed at each stage of the process.

Fill in Figure 5.1. Think about:

- things you do
- whether you do them alone or with other people
- why you like it that way.

The first five activities have been written in for you. Think of another five activities yourself.

Activity	By myself or with others		Why?
Doing the washing up	Myself ○	Others ○	
Painting a picture	Myself ○	Others ○	
Doing homework	Myself ○	Others ○	
Taking five children on a trip	Myself ○	Others ○	
Redecorating the living room	Myself ○	Others ○	
_____	Myself ○	Others ○	
_____	Myself ○	Others ○	
_____	Myself ○	Others ○	
_____	Myself ○	Others ○	
_____	Myself ○	Others ○	

Figure 5.1 Activities of working with others (Clark 2010)

Leadership – working with others

As a work-based facilitator you will be expected to take on a leadership role, facilitating the learning experience, but also leading others to ensure that learning opportunities are provided. It is important that you have an understanding of the people that you work with and understand how you use power, influence and authority:

- *Power* is the ability to influence others.
- *Influence* is the process of getting A to do something or think something that A would not have done otherwise.
- *Authority* is the right to use power over the behaviour of others. It is the legitimate power that goes with roles and position.

The facilitator role has a position of power, resource power, expert power and personal power, so all in all you are a very powerful person, who can influence greatly students' behaviour by using this authority.

You will also need to demonstrate leadership qualities. Studies of chief executives have concluded that leaders demonstrate the following factors:

- ability to work with a wide range of people
- early overall responsibility for important tasks
- strong achievement goals
- experience of leading a group
- wide experience of several functions.

What leadership qualities do you exhibit? How do you relate to others and what do you need to improve to become a better leader? The following activity (Clark 2010) will assist you to answer these questions.

ACTIVITY 5.5

The behaviours listed in Figure 5.2 below are essential to relating to others. Rate yourself on these behaviours, using the following scale:

1	2	3	4	5	6	7	8	9
Very Weak	Moderately Weak		Adequate		Moderately Strong			Very Strong

Note: a rating of 5 means that you would consider yourself a resource person (if only minimally so). That is, in a relationship or group, you would be a giver rather than just a receiver.

1 _____ **Feelings:** I am not afraid to deal directly with emotion, whether it is my own or others'. I allow myself to feel and give expression to what I feel.

2 _____ **Initiative:** In my relationships I act rather than react by going out and contacting others without waiting to be contacted.

3 _____ **Respect:** I express that I am for others even if I do not necessarily approve of what they do.

4 _____ **Genuineness:** I do not hide behind roles or facades. I let others know where I stand.

5 _____ **Concreteness:** I am not vague when I speak to others. I do not beat around the bush in that I deal with concrete experience and behaviour.

6 _____ **Immediacy:** I deal openly and directly with others. I know where I stand with others and they know where they stand with me.

7 _____ **Empathy:** I see the world through the eyes of others by listening to cues, both verbal and non-verbal, and I respond to these cues.

8 _____ **Confrontation:** I challenge others with responsibility and with care. I do not use confrontation to punish.

9 _____ **Self-disclosure:** I let others know the person inside, but I am not exhibitionistic. I am open without being a secret-reveller or secret-searcher.

10 _____ **Self-exploration:** I examine my life style and behaviours and want others to help me to do so. I am open to change.

Figure 5.2 Working with others rating scale (Clark 2010)

Scoring

There are no correct or incorrect scores. This assessment simply shows you where you stand in your relations with others. Your goal should be to work on the lowest scorings of the 10 behaviours.

Also, have one or two others rate you so that you can get an outside view of yourself as to whether you are projecting yourself to others as you believe you are.

Competencies of working with others

Table 5.1 (US Coast Guard 2004) outlines the competencies you should develop to ensure effective group working.

Table 5.1 Competencies of effective group working

Competency	Behaviours
Influencing others	• Motivate others to achieve desired outcomes by directing, coaching and delegating as the situation requires • Recognise the importance of building professional relationships • Develop networks of contacts and colleagues • Establish rapport with key players • Empower others by delegating power and responsibility and hold them accountable • Gain cooperation and commitment from others
Respect for others and diversity management	• Understand and support the commitment to respect for every individual in the workplace • Recognise and promote the value of diversity • Foster an environment that supports diverse individuals and perspectives, fairness, dignity, compassion and creativity in the workplace
Looking out for others	• Recognise the needs and abilities of others, particularly subordinates • Ensure fair and equitable treatment • Provide opportunities for professional development • Recognise and reward performance • Support and assist others in professional and personal situations
Effective communication	• Learn to express facts and ideas succinctly and logically • Be an active and supportive listener • Encourage open exchange of ideas • Communicate face-to-face when possible • Write clearly and concisely • Speak effectively before an audience • Distinguish between personal and official communication situations and act accordingly
Group dynamics	• Build commitment, pride, team spirit and strong relationships • Recognise and contribute to group efforts • Foster group identity and cooperation • Motivate and guide others toward goal accomplishment • Consider and respond to others' needs and capabilities
Leadership theory	• Study and understand different leadership theories and styles • Work with subordinates to develop their leadership knowledge and skills • Adapt leadership approaches to meet varying situations including crises
Mentoring	• Assist others in their development by sharing your experience and knowledge • Provide feedback to others on their leadership and career development • Help others identify professional goals, strengths and areas for improvement

Source: US Coast Guard (2004)

The unit on Supporting Learning in the Workplace, plus the supplementary learning materials on Communication will give you more information on developing your communication skills. You may also find them helpful in supporting your student.

Dealing with conflict

> **ACTIVITY 5.6**
>
> Conflict occurs at times between and within teams. This activity will assist you in considering what strategies you use and need to develop to deal with conflict.
>
> How do you think you deal with conflict?
>
> Answer the questions on this website:
>
> http://www.sideroad.com/Leadership/conflict-style.html
>
> Tick which style best describes how you approach conflict in the workplace:
>
> * avoid
> * compete
> * accommodate
> * compromise
> * collaborate.
>
> What are your strengths in dealing with conflict?
>
> What aspects can you identify that require development in how you deal with conflict?

Working with others is not without its difficulties. Problems and at times conflict can occur. It is important that these are resolved to ensure effective and efficient working.

Resolving conflict

Each side should come together and work cooperatively on the issues and where necessary have someone to act as a facilitator.

The process would then require the following steps:

* Gather information: identify key issues without making accusations; focus on what the issues are, not who did what; do not accuse, find fault or call names.
* Each party states their position and how it has affected them; others listen attentively and respectfully without interruption.
* Each party, in turn, repeats or describes as best they can the other's position *to* the listener's satisfaction. Parties try to view the issue from other points of view beside the two conflicting ones.
* Parties brainstorm to find the middle ground, a point of balance, creative solutions, etc.
* Each side volunteers what he or she can do to resolve the conflict or solve the problem.
* A formal agreement is drawn up with agreed-upon actions for both parties.
* A procedure is identified, should disagreement arise.
* Progress is monitored.
* Progress is rewarded or celebrated.

Each party in collaborative conflict resolution should feel empowered to speak their mind, feel listened to and feel that they are a critical part of the solution. So, also, each is obligated to respect and listen to others, try to understand their point of view and actively work toward a mutual decision.

If the conflict cannot be resolved in this manner, mediation by a third, neutral party (as in peer mediation) or arbitration (enforced resolution by a neutral authority) are options.

Education is an excellent setting to learn problem-solving and conflict resolution strategies. Whether the conflict is a classroom real-life simulation activity or an on-going emotional experience, learning ways to resolve issues and collaboratively work through responses and solutions will teach you skills that can be applied in other settings. Friends School of Minnesota (2012) believes that it can help you to:

- accept differences
- recognise mutual interests
- improve persuasion skills
- improve listening skills
- break the reactive cycle or routine
- learn to disagree without animosity
- build confidence in recognising win-win solutions
- recognise/admit to/process anger and other emotions
- solve problems!

Negotiating strategies

In order to resolve conflict, at times you will require negotiation strategies and will hope for win-win outcomes that have been described above. Unfortunately, some opponents will attempt to win at all costs. Beware of the following negotiating strategies:

Fait accompli strategy: the fait accompli strategy is a risky one. Basically, one side does whatever it wants and expects the other side to accept the terms and the outcome.

Standard practice strategy: the 'standard practice' claim infers that what is being suggested is acceptable because it is 'standard practice'. This strategy is another reason why doing your homework is important. If you are negotiating in an area that may be unfamiliar to you, be sure you research any 'standard practice' claims before agreeing to them.

Deadline strategy: time can be a powerful weapon in a negotiation. If the other side knows your deadlines they may delay giving you a draft (and possibly throw in a few changes) until the last minute to gain the advantage. The closer you are to your deadlines, the more concessions you're likely to make. Therefore, it is important to set a deadline which you are happy with.

Decoy strategy: the decoy issue is often used by politicians. This strategy involves inflating the importance of a minor issue to mask the importance of a larger issue or a hidden agenda. If the other side concedes what they have made you believe is a major issue, but what is for them a minor one, they will then expect you to concede on one of your truly important issues. Again, doing your homework will give you an edge in knowing the industry value of various issues.

Faking withdrawal strategy: faking withdrawal from the deal in favour of a competitor is another strategy of which to be wary. Its purpose is to gain a concession, usually a significant one, by pretending to entertain another offer such as one from your competition. If you catch the other party in this strategy, it's probably best to call their bluff and end the negotiations in favour of going elsewhere, perhaps to their competition.

Good guy/bad guy strategy: this approach is easy to spot. A common scenario may go something like this: one of the negotiators on the other side is hard core (definitely not win-win minded) in his/her approach. This strategy may even involve the 'bad guy' throwing a temper tantrum. Then, when the bad guy steps out for a few minutes, the good guy half of the negotiating team makes an offer in a less threatening manner. If the other side has resorted to this strategy, it may be best to call them on it or consider terminating the negotiations.

Limited authority strategy: the limited authority strategy involves the other side trying to make concessions by claiming they don't have the authority to make concessions on their own. If the other side claims that they do not have the authority to lower the price, but instead need to call a manager, you should halt negotiations with that person and only resume talks with a representative who has the authority to truly negotiate.

Salami strategy: the salami technique is used to gain concessions piece by piece. The basic premise is this: instead of trying to grab the whole salami, cut off thin slices over time. The result is gaining the whole or a good portion of the salami without the other side realising it (Thomas *et al.* 2006).

Assertiveness

Have you been in a situation where you wanted to say something, but didn't, in order to avoid having a row? Or perhaps you got so angry that you had a violent outburst and regretted it afterwards? Then assertive communication would have helped.

Lack of assertiveness can affect your relationships and quality of life; there are a number of ways in which you can begin to assert yourself.

What is assertiveness?

Assertiveness is an attitude and a way of relating to the outside world, backed up by a set of skills. You need to see yourself as being of worth. This goes hand in hand with you valuing others equally and respecting their right to an opinion. Assertiveness ensures that you are not hurt, used or abused.

ACTIVITY 5.7

Would you describe yourself as assertive?

Explain your answer.

In what situations in work do you find it difficult to be assertive?

1

2

3

4

What do you currently do in these situations?

1

2

3

4

Many people find it difficult to communicate honestly, directly and openly with other people. There are two other main ways of relating to others: being passive or being aggressive.

Assertiveness involves the following:

- being clear about what you feel, what you need and how it can be achieved
- being able to communicate calmly without attacking another person
- saying 'yes' when you want to and saying 'no' when you mean 'no' (rather than agreeing to do something just to please someone else)
- deciding on, and sticking to, clear boundaries – being happy to defend your position, even if it provokes conflict
- being confident about handling conflict if it occurs
- understanding how to negotiate if two people want different outcomes
- being able to talk openly about yourself and being able to listen to others
- having confident, open body language
- being able to give and receive positive and negative feedback
- having a positive, optimistic outlook.

Passivity

Passive modes of communication are adopted when someone doesn't know how to express themselves assertively; they tend to resort to these in an attempt to punish or undermine the other person. They may play games, use sarcasm, give in resentfully, or remain silent at their own cost.

Aggression

It is sometimes said about assertive behaviour that it involves being aggressive. Assertiveness involves clear, calm thinking and respectful negotiation, where each person is entitled to their opinion. Aggression involves bottling up feelings, which eventually explode, leaving no room for communication.

Some people think that being assertive is about being selfish; it is in fact the opposite. Assertiveness is about acknowledging all opinions as important. An assertive attitude says 'I matter and you do too'. Learning how to express yourself assertively can seem difficult at first, but you can develop the skills of assertiveness.

Body language

Part of assertiveness is open, secure body language. The way that you present yourself has an impact on how you are perceived and treated. Passive body language would be the classic 'victim' stance of hunched shoulders and avoidance of eye contact, while an aggressive stance is one with clenched fists, glaring eyes and intrusive body language.

Assertive people generally stand upright but in a relaxed manner, looking people calmly in the eyes, with open hands. A good first step to becoming more assertive is to consider your own body language through role play.

ACTIVITY 5.8

With a friend, or in front of a mirror, try different types of posture and body language as you imagine being the aggressor, the victim and finally an assertive person. Your friend can play the opposite role of passive versus aggressive and so on. Finally, see what it feels like to change from being in a passive/aggressive stance to using assertive body language. Just standing in a confident, calm way can feel empowering.

Communication

Clear communication is an important part of assertiveness. This is where you show:

- knowledge – you are able to understand and summarise the situation
- feelings – you can explain your feelings about the situation
- needs – you are able to explain clearly what you want or need, giving your reasons and any benefits to the other party.

Assertive communication

It isn't 'what you say' that counts, but it is the 'way you say it' that matters. It helps to:

- be honest with yourself about your own feelings
- keep calm and stick to the point
- be clear, specific and direct

- if you meet objections, keep repeating your message whilst also listening to the other's point of view; try to offer alternative solutions if you can; ask, if you are unsure about something
- if the other person tries to create a diversion, point this out calmly and repeat your message
- use appropriate body language
- always respect the rights and point of view of the other person.

ACTIVITY 5.9

With a friend, practise being assertive in certain work situations, such as refusing to accept additional work or having to give constructive criticism to a colleague. Explain the scenario to your friend. Using role play, go through the situation, making your points clearly, with your friend responding as the other person.

Afterwards, ask your friend to tell you what went well and where you could make improvements.

Try the situation again. Then swap roles to see the other person's perspective.

Once you have practised being more assertive, think through your new techniques before entering a situation that requires assertiveness. Imagine your body language and work out how to deliver your message clearly. Imagine how you will react to any possible responses.

(Adapted from BUPA's Health Information Team April 2011)

The learning materials on Communication listed in this unit's bibliography will give you more information on developing your skills. You may also find them helpful in supporting your student.

ACTIVITY 5.10

Look back on your situations where you found it difficult to be assertive and outline an assertive response that you could try.

1
2
3
4

Developing strategies for effective working

To work effectively with others in the workplace you and your student must develop strategies for effective working. These include the following:

- set priorities and manage your time to meet deadlines
- set and achieve goals
- get over your internal barriers when putting your goals and plans into action
- effectively organise your daily actions
- uncover better options
- work in a team or build one
- prevent burnout.

Conclusion

This unit has given you a brief introduction into the importance of working with others in the workplace. It has tried to stimulate your thinking about the groups that you work with and their purpose and function. The activities have been designed to assist you in using the theory provided to relate it to your own situation and context. The literature about working with others is extensive and may be found in most management texts, so you may find it useful to read more widely on the topics mentioned in this unit.

References

Belbin, M. (2010) *Management Teams: Why They Succeed or Fail*. 3rd edition. Butterworth-Heinemann.

BUPA Health Information Team (2011) *Improving Assertiveness*. http://hcd2.bupa.co.uk/fact_sheets/html/improving_assertiveness.html

CAIPE (2012) *Definition and Principles of Interprofessional Education*. www.caipe.org.uk/resources

Clark, D. (2010) *Leadership: Working with Others*. www.nwlink.com/~donclark/leader/behavor.html

Friends School of Minnesota (2012) *Conflict Resolution Training Manual*. www.fsmn.org/about/our-approach/conflict-resolution/cr-manual

Key Skills Support Programme (2005) *Working with Others*. http://archive.excellencegateway.org.uk/page.aspx?o=224137

Porteus, A. (2012) *Roles People Play in Groups*. *http://*www.stanford.edu/group/resed/resed/staffresources/RM/training/grouproles.html

Thomas, P., Sattler, E. D. and Doniek, M. S. (2006) *Fitness Management*. Courtney Hadden.

Tuckman, B. (1965) Developmental Sequence in Small Groups. *Psychological Bulletin* 63: 384–99.

Tuckman, B. and Jensen, M. (1977) Stages of Small Group Development. *Group and Organizational Studies* 2: 419–27.

US Coast Guard (2004) *Competencies of Working with Others*. www.au.af.mil/au/awc/awcgate/uscg/ldr_comp_2004.pdf

Bibliography

Adler, R. B. and Elmhorst, J. M. (1999) *Communicating at Work: Principles and Practices for Business and the Professions*. McGraw Hill.

Blundel, R. (1998) *Effective Business Communication*. Prentice Hall.

Clampitt, P. G. (2005) *Communicating for Managerial Effectiveness*. Sage.

Cole, K. (1993) *Crystal Clear Communication*. Prentice Hall.

DeVito, J. (1990) *The Elements of Public Speaking*. Harper & Row.

Dickson, D. (1999) Barriers to Communication. In Long, A. (ed.), *Interaction for Practice in Community Nursing*. Macmillan.

Ellis, R. (2002) *Communication Skills: Stepladders to Success for the Professional*. Intellect Books.

Gallagher, K., McLelland, B. and Swales, C. (1998) Business Skills: An Active Learning Approach. In Hartley, P. and Bruckman, C. G. (2002), *Business Communication*. Routledge.

Goleman, D. (1996) *Emotional Intelligence*. Bloomsbury.

Goman, C. K. (2002) Cross-cultural Business Practices. *Communication World* 19: 22–25.

Hamilton, C. and Parker, C. (1990) Communicating for Results. In Hargie, O., Dickson, D. and Tourish, D. (2004), op cit.

Hargie, O., Dickson, D. and Tourish, D. (2004) *Communication Skills for Effective Management*. Palgrave Macmillan.

Hartley, P. and Bruckman, C. G. (2002) *Business Communication*. Routledge.

Hill, L. (1996) *Building Effective One-on-One Work Relationships*. Harvard Business School Technical Notes.

Kotter, J. P. (1982) What Effective General Managers Really Do? *Harvard Business Review* 60: 156–167.

McClure, P. (2005) *Reflection on Practice*. www.science.ulster.ac.uk/nursing/mentorship/docs/learning/reflectiononpractice.pdf

Nichols, R. G. and Stevens, L. A. (1990) Listening to People. *Harvard Business Review* 68: 95–102.

Rasberry, R. W. and Lemoine, L. F. (1986) *Effective Managerial Communication*. MA Kent.

Spitzberg, B. H. (1994) The Dark Side of Incompetence. In Adler, R. B. and Elmhorst, J. M. (1999), op cit.

Stewart, J. and Logan, C. (1998) Together: Communicating Interpersonally. In Hargie, O., Dickson, D. and Tourish, D. (2004), op cit.

Stiff, J. B., Hale, J. L., Garlick, R. and Rogan, R. G. (1990) Effect of Cue Incongruence and Social Normative Influences on Individual Judgements of Honesty and Deceit. *Southern Speech Communication Journal* 55: 206–29.

Tourish, D. and Hargie, O. (2004) *Key Issues in Organisational Communication*. Routledge.

Venn, P. (2005) www.science.ulster.ac.uk/nursing/mentorship/docs/learning/CommsSkillsV2.pdf

Wells, G. (1986) *How to Communicate*. McGraw-Hill.

Wertheim, E. G. (2005) www.science.ulster.ac.uk/nursing/mentorship/docs/learning/ CommsSkillsV2.pdf

Wilson, G. and Nias, D. (1999) in Guerrero, L. and DeVito, J. (eds) *The Nonverbal Communication Reader: Classic and Contemporary Readings*. Waveland Press.

Diversity in the workplace

Introduction

We are living in an era of rapid social and technological change. These changes are taking place at different rates across the globe. The pace of change in some countries has accelerated with economic growth and development. As for the advances in science and technology, these are making it possible for us to live our lives in ways we want to and they influence where we live and affect everything that is associated with living in urban as well as rural environments. Work-based facilitators need to acknowledge the impact of the diverse nature of students learning in the workplace.

Aim of the unit

The aim of this unit is to assist work-based facilitators in understanding the dimensions of difference that impact upon student learning during work-based placements.

Outcomes of the unit

At the end of this unit you will be able to:

1 identify the diverse needs of individuals involved in learning in the workplace
2 maximise the individual's potential for learning in the workplace
3 work with a range of people from different backgrounds.

Nature of diversity

In Britain today, we live side by side with people from different ethnic, cultural, social and religious backgrounds. We are becoming increasingly aware of the fact that we live in a multi-ethnic and multicultural society. Depending upon where we live or work, or which services we access in the community, we have probably seen changes to our communities over a period of time. We are increasingly aware of the differences and similarities among ourselves, and others, in relation to age, gender, ethnicity, culture, religious beliefs and practices, social and economic status, educational and occupational backgrounds, disability, sexual orientation, health and the impact of illness.

Directgov (2012a) argues that there must be no unfair discrimination on the basis of age, disability, gender, marital status, sexual orientation, religion or belief, race, colour, nationality, ethnic or national origin, or (in Northern Ireland) community background, working pattern, employment status, gender identity (transgender), caring responsibility or trade union membership.

In everyday life, we may find our long-held ideas about ourselves as well as others challenged when we encounter people from diverse cultural backgrounds. Our levels of understanding about other cultures may vary. In some instances our observations may be superficial and our knowledge less developed, based on media representations or limited encounters with people from different ethnic and cultural backgrounds. In other cases, it may be that through personal and professional contact we have been able to establish over time an understanding of others from diverse backgrounds. In modern urban environments, it is likely that cultural diversity is an obvious reality for all of us, yet we must acknowledge our level of awareness and sensitivity, or lack of it, in order to demonstrate our respect for others.

ACTIVITY 6.1

Think of a time when you felt excluded (this could be a social occasion at work or a meeting). What were your

- thoughts?
- feelings?
- physical reactions?
- behaviour?

Think of a time when you felt included (again, it could be a social occasion at work or a meeting). What were your

- thoughts?
- feelings?
- physical reactions?
- behaviour?

What are the benefits of encouraging students to feel your workplace is inclusive?

Valuing diversity is an essential aspect of living and working in a multicultural society. As a work-based educator you need to become aware of the cultural influences on students' behaviour and translate that awareness into a culturally congruent placement experience (Mary Seacole Centre 2012).

Stereotyping others in terms of ethnicity, spirituality, age, gender, disability and sexual orientation can give rise to negative and positive stereotypes, which can lead to prejudice and discrimination. Therefore, you need to develop the knowledge, skills and attitudinal responses to meet the needs of students undertaking work-based placement with respect, sensitivity and the competence required to ensure effective learning occurs.

Legislation

Discrimination against members of diverse groups, such as on the grounds of sex, gender, gender reassignment, age, race, ethnic or national origins, colour, marital status, sexuality, family responsibility, disability or impairment, or religious or other beliefs is not allowed in the United Kingdom.

Equality Act 2010

The Act replaced a number of anti-discrimination laws covering England, Scotland and Wales with a single Act, covering discrimination on various grounds including disability, gender reassignment, pregnancy and maternity, race, religion or belief, sex and sexual orientation. The Act covers direct discrimination, discrimination by association, discrimination by perception, indirect discrimination, harassment, victimisation and positive action.

The Equality Act 2010 covers principles of several Acts referred to later within this unit, e.g. Carers (Equal) Opportunities Act 2004, Disability Discrimination Acts of 1995 and 2005

(Department for Work and Pensions 2005) and Employment Equality (Sexual Orientation) Regulations 2003, whilst extending their provision as outlined in the previous paragraph.

Disability Discrimination (Northern Ireland) Order 2006

This legislation covering Northern Ireland extended coverage provided by the Disability Discrimination Act 1995 (see below), by having a more extensive definition of disability and providing wider areas of protection, e.g. in private clubs, job advertisements and transport. The Order also brought public authorities' functions into the scope of the legislation.

Disability Discrimination Act 1995

This legislation defines disability as a 'physical or mental impairment that has a long-term adverse impact on someone's ability to carry out normal day-to-day duties' and outlaws discrimination on the grounds of disability in employment, education, the provision of goods and services and transport. Employers and the providers of goods and services must put in place reasonable adjustments to meet the specific request of a disabled person that will facilitate their participation.

Disability Discrimination Act 2005

This legislation extended the provisions of the 1995 Act by extending the definition of disability and ending the requirement for mental illness to be clinically recognised before considered an impairment and made various amendments covering transport, rented dwellings and private clubs, as well as bringing any public authorities not covered by the 1995 Act within the scope of the 2005 Act and placing a duty on public authorities to promote equality of opportunity for disabled people.

Defining diversity

ACTIVITY 6.2
What do you understand by the term diversity?

Most definitions of diversity are, according to the Royal College of Nursing (2006a), based on the following ideas:

- A person's diversity adds value to the organisation if managed effectively.
- Diversity includes almost all ways in which people differ, such as education and sexual orientation, as well as the more obvious ones of gender, ethnicity and disability.
- Diversity has as its primary concern organisational culture and the working environment.

Here are some key terms used in relation to diversity, based on the work of Fernandez and Fernandez (2012) and the Honolulu Community College (2012):

- Culture refers to norms and practices of a particular group that are learned and shared and guide thinking, decisions, and actions.
- Cultural values are individuals' desirable or preferred way of acting or knowing something that is sustained over a period of time and which governs actions or decisions.
- Culturally diverse support refers to the need to provide culturally appropriate student support that incorporates individuals' cultural values, beliefs and practices including sensitivity to the environment from which the individual comes and to which the individual may ultimately return.

- Ethnocentrism is the perception that one's own way is best when viewing the world (Geiger and Davidhizar 2008). Our perspective is the standard by which all other perspectives are measured and held to scrutiny.
- Ethnic relates to group identification, with large groups of people being classified according to common traits or customs.
- Race refers to the different varieties of humans assumed by some people to exist, based on the discredited typological model of human variation.
- Discrimination is differential treatment of an individual due to minority status, both actual and perceived; e.g. 'We just aren't equipped to serve people like that.'
- Stereotyping is generalising about a person while ignoring the presence of individual difference; e.g. 'She's like that because she's Asian – all Asians are non-verbal.'
- Cultural blindness occurs when differences are ignored and one proceeds as though differences did not exist; e.g. 'There's no need to worry about a person's culture – if you're a sensitive teacher, you do okay.'
- Cultural imposition is the belief that everyone should conform to the majority; e.g. 'We know what's best for you; if you don't like it, you can go elsewhere.'

All interpersonal communication contains the possibility of ambiguity and misunderstanding (Royal College of Nursing 2006b). The possibilities of misunderstanding and poor communication become much greater when we communicate across a cultural boundary. Experience routinely makes us anxious about the appropriateness and adequacy of our behaviour in cross-cultural contexts. Consequently, at the outset it is important that we explicitly recognise the normality of such anxieties and the challenge faced by us all in operating effectively in a multi-ethnic context.

ACTIVITY 6.3

How much does your workplace value diversity?

What is the evidence that diversity is addressed in your workplace?

List the action(s) you need to take in relation to meeting the diverse needs of students undertaking a work-based placement? (This may be useful to include in your portfolio.)

Nature of diversity

This next part of the unit examines the nature of diversity in relation to work-based learning by identifying some of the features of diversity that result in diverse student needs within contemporary society. These features include those described below.

Dyslexia

Mitchell (2012) provides extensive information about dyslexia. She states that the word dyslexia comes from the Greek, meaning 'difficulty with words', and encompasses a wide variety of features. There are many positive aspects to being dyslexic, including being creative, being able to think multi-dimensionally (that is, in 3D), or in pictures, thinking laterally and being good at solving problems. Being dyslexic is not just about misspelling words or mixing up letters. It can also include difficulty in organising thoughts and differentiating between left and right, and problems with short-term memory.

Like all of us, dyslexics have their own individual mixture of strengths and weaknesses. Some may find things harder or easier than others, and may also have developed different ways of dealing with their dyslexia. Dyslexics may really struggle in education as reading and writing are the main skills that are valued. Children who are dyslexic have often been made to feel stupid at school, and may never have had the chance to find or show their creative skills.

People may be born dyslexic, or become dyslexic if they experience brain damage. The exact causes of dyslexia are not known; however, it is known that dyslexics process their thoughts differently to non-dyslexic people. About 3 per cent to 10 per cent of the general population is dyslexic, and approximately 2 per cent of UK undergraduate students are dyslexic. The exact number is not known; not everyone knows if they are dyslexic, and some people don't tell anyone they are dyslexic because they don't feel any need to, or because they feel ashamed. It is likely that you know someone who is dyslexic.

Some say that people with dyslexia are often able to think and work differently, which means they produce innovative and creative solutions to problems. For example, an exhibition-support company based in Birmingham prefers to employ dyslexics because they bring an 'added benefit' to business by heightened ability to 'think outside the box'.

Dyslexics may be lateral thinkers, who are able to come up with unusual solutions to problems. It is said that dyslexics are able to experience multiple views of the world, and will often see letters in three dimensions. For example, Lord Rogers is a famous architect and dyslexic, who has designed the Pompidou centre in Paris amongst other buildings. Thus it can be seen that, with these qualities, dyslexics can excel in all sorts of occupations. Some actors are dyslexic, such as Bob Hoskins and Susan Hampshire. Some dyslexics are successful in business, such as Richard Branson, Chairman of Virgin Group, Richard Wray, Virgin Mobile Chief Executive, Guy Hands, financier, and Neil Holloway, Chief Executive of Microsoft UK.

Some dyslexics experience difficulties such as leaving letters out in words, reversing letters or letters appearing to move on the page. They may leave words out in sentences, or put them in a different order. Some people don't show any of the things that most people associate with being dyslexic, for example, they may be good at spelling.

They may have difficulty in remembering things, such as telephone numbers and PIN numbers. They may have difficulty in organising thoughts in sequence, and giving or following instructions, or keeping diary appointments. They may also find it hard to remember which is left and which is right. These problems can be made worse if the person feels stressed.

Dyslexics may have problems in copying information down and making notes, such as in lectures or meetings, because they are slow at writing, or they have to think how a word is spelled. They may have difficulty organising their thoughts when writing reports or essays and, if they rely on their spell-checkers, they may sometimes choose an inappropriate word. Students may be taught adaptive strategies to use to deal with these difficulties. Graphical ways of organising notes and ideas such as mind maps are often very successful. However, students may need help in transferring their adaptive strategies to a new environment, such as work.

Bournemouth University (2012) provides an overview of how dyslexia can manifest itself in students:

- discrepancy between general abilities and language skills (language skills not learnt subliminally – e.g. spelling not 'caught' by reading)
- variation in performance – good day/bad day
- difficulty generalising and applying new rules
- poor short term memory:
  - difficulty holding large chunks of auditory information long enough to process it into long-term memory – so following lectures can be difficult
  - difficulty retaining information that has been read – so may need to read the same thing several times, resulting in slower reading
  - difficulty remembering facts or new terminology
  - may misplace items, forget names/telephone numbers, instructions
  - difficulty with rote learning of tables, number facts or procedural sequences
- short concentration span
- difficulty in taking part in discussion
- taking longer to process information
- may lack general knowledge due to lack of reading ability
- may experience difficulty in feeding back information due to the inability to structure and remember information

- coordination difficulties
- poor organisational skills
- may have difficulty remembering and managing time or organising coursework and materials – so may miss classes and deadlines
- poor sequencing skills
- difficulty structuring essays; may repeat information
- difficulty with alphabetic order, months of year, seasons, tables, lists of instructions
- issues with reading:
  - will require in advance anything that needs to be read aloud, e.g. scripts, etc
  - because of retention problems, may read more slowly
  - may have difficulty tracking text due to moving/glaring print – may lose place
  - difficulty decoding unfamiliar words
  - difficulty with comprehension and therefore summarising
  - difficulty translating worded problems into numerical tasks
  - may reverse numbers read from calculator
- issues with writing:
  - poor spelling, grammar, punctuation and handwriting
  - word-finding problems can interrupt flow of ideas
  - simultaneous handling of sequential expression of ideas, word retrieval, grammar, spelling and typing/handwriting difficult
  - written work may not adequately reflect understanding and ideas
  - copying from board/overhead projector is difficult
  - may not be able to read own notes afterwards
  - may reverse letters and numbers
- pronunciation/articulation and word retrieval difficulties
- low self esteem; lack of confidence; frustration; anxiety; embarrassment
- tiredness – brought on by intense concentration.

Work-based facilitators should take note of the various ways in which dyslexia can present and provide relevant support for dyslexic students, which will be considered later in this unit.

ACTIVITY 6.4

Are there aspects of your practice that would disadvantage a student with dyslexia?

What action could you take to address this?

What organisational changes would be needed? (This could be useful to include in your portfolio.)

Ethnicity and culture

The Mary Seacole Centre (2012) states that the word culture has been used to describe many aspects of social life. As a result, the label 'culture' has been attached to many expressions of social life, food, arts, clothing, music and practices. Culture has also been used to distinguish social groups in terms of language, religious beliefs, education and other factors. Hofstede *et al.* (2010) have suggested that culture can be defined as 'the interactive aggregate of common characteristics that influence a human group's responses to its environment'. This definition makes a clear association between humans and their environment, which is established as an important interactive relationship, each affecting the other.

Purnell and Paulanka (2008) have defined culture as 'the totality of socially transmitted behavioural patterns, arts, beliefs, values, customs, lifeways, and all other products of human work and thought characteristics of a population of people that guide their worldview and decision making'. This definition captures the essence of culture. The transmission is from people to people, and is intergenerational.

Elsewhere, Geiger and Davidhizar (2008) define culture as 'a patterned behavioural response that develops over time as a result of imprinting the mind through social and religious structures and intellectual and artistic manifestations'. This definition suggests the action or behavioural orientation of cultural influences. Building on this definition, they advance explanations about culture. Culture is shaped and in turn acts as a means of shaping our thinking and doing.

Ethnicity is a common term used in health and related sciences, and most definitions include references to place of origin, or ancestry, skin colour, cultural heritage, religion and language. Ethnicity denotes a sense of kinship, group solidarity and a common culture. According to Cliffs Notes (2012), ethnicity refers to shared cultural practices and perspectives, and distinctions that set apart one group of people from another. That is, ethnicity is a shared cultural heritage. The most common characteristics distinguishing various ethnic groups are ancestry, a sense of history, language, religion and forms of dress. Ethnic differences are not inherited; they are learned. We all belong to ethnic groups even though the term 'ethnic' is often incorrectly used in a short-hand way to only refer to individuals from black and minority backgrounds. Individuals may perceive themselves as belonging to particular ethnic groups and identify themselves with people with whom they feel they share a common sense of identity. Thus, there are objective and subjective facets to ethnicity.

The objective facet includes factual and observable characteristics such as ancestry, place of birth, cultural factors, religion and language – these can be used as objective indicators to examine the concept of ethnicity. The subjective element is important to the individual's perception and identification of his/her ethnicity, and the group that he/she belongs to. In this instance, the individual may assign himself/herself an ethnic identity, an ethnic group affiliation. However, such assignment is a matter of choice and preference, and individuals may equally choose not to state their ethnicity. Ethnic identity is part of cultural identity; it is an interpretation by the individual and is subjective. In addition, Culley *et al.* (2009) believe that ethnic identity is overlaid with a range of variables, including gender, age, socio-economic and professional identities, each of which may be more or less significant in any specific situation, at any specific moment. When the sense of ethnic identity is strong, individuals maintain solidarity, ethnic group values, beliefs, language and culture.

Clark (2010) highlights the importance of realising that we allow our past experiences to change the meaning of the message. Our culture, background and bias can be good as they allow us to use our past experiences to understand something new; it is when they change the meaning of the message that they then interfere with the communication process. Work-based facilitators need to be aware that students from different ethnic backgrounds may bring different perspectives to a placement. In addition, there is diversity within any group, and one should be careful about generalising certain attributes/behaviours to all members of an ethnic group.

ACTIVITY 6.5

Are there aspects of your practice that would disadvantage a student on a cultural or ethnic basis?

What action could you take to address this?

What changes would be needed within your organisation? (This could be useful to include in your portfolio.)

Religion and spirituality

The BBC (2012) provides an overview of a range of religions and beliefs, including:

- Atheism: Atheists are people who do not believe in a god or gods (or other immaterial beings), or who believe that these concepts are not meaningful. Some atheists put it more firmly and believe that god or gods do not exist.

- Buddhism: Buddhism is a tradition that focuses on personal spiritual development. Buddhists strive for a deep insight into the true nature of life and do not worship gods or deities. At the heart of the Buddha's teaching lie The Four Noble Truths and The Eightfold Path which lead the Buddhist towards the path of Enlightenment. The Buddha taught that the human tendency is to avoid the difficult truths of life and that this in turn leads to suffering. By enabling the mind to be at peace through meditation, a human being can confront reality and overcome hatred and craving.

- Christianity: Christianity is the world's biggest religion, with about 2.1 billion followers worldwide. It is based on the teachings of Jesus Christ who lived in the Holy Land 2,000 years ago. Christians believe that there is only one God, whom they call *Father* as Jesus Christ taught them. Christians recognise Jesus as the Son of God who was sent to save mankind from death and sin. Jesus Christ taught that he was the Son of God. His teachings can be summarised, briefly, as the love of God and love of one's neighbour. Christians believe in justification by faith – that through their belief in Jesus as the Son of God, and in his death and resurrection, they can have a right relationship with God whose forgiveness was given once and for all through the death of Jesus Christ.

- Hinduism: Hinduism originated over 3,000 years ago. Hinduism claims to have many founders, teachers and prophets who claim first-hand experience of God. When Hindus promote the idea of spirituality as a principle rather than a personality, they call this *Brahman*. The gods of the Hindu faith represent different expressions of Brahman. Different Hindu communities may have their own divinities whom they worship, but these are simply different ways of approaching the Ultimate.

- Islam: Islam began in Arabia and was revealed to humanity by the Prophet Muhammad (peace be upon him). Those who follow Islam are called Muslims. Muslims believe that there is only one God. The Arabic word for God is *Allah*. Muslims have six main beliefs:
  - Belief in Allah as the one and only God.
  - Belief in angels.
  - Belief in the holy books.
  - Belief in the Prophets:
    - e.g. Adam, Ibrahim (Abraham), Musa (Moses), Dawud (David), Isa (Jesus).
    - Muhammad (peace be upon him) is the final prophet.
  - Belief in the Day of Judgement:
    - This is the day when the life of every human being will be assessed to decide whether they go to heaven or hell.
  - Belief in Predestination:
    - i.e. belief that Allah has already decided what will happen.
    - Muslims believe that this doesn't stop human beings from making free choices.

- Jehovah's Witnesses: Jehovah's Witnesses are members of a Christian-based religious movement probably best known for their door-to-door evangelical work. Jehovah's Witnesses see themselves as a worldwide brotherhood that transcends national boundaries and national and ethnic loyalties. They believe that, since Christ proclaimed that his kingdom was no part of the world and refused to accept a temporal crown, they too must keep separate from the world and refrain from political involvement.

- Judaism: Judaism is around 3,500 years old. Jews believe that there is only one God and that the Jewish People were specially chosen to receive God's guidance. Jews believe that there is a single God who not only created the universe, but with whom every Jew can have an individual and personal relationship. They believe that God continues to work in the world, affecting everything that people do.

- Rastafari: Rastafari is a young religion. It developed in Jamaica in the 1930s following the coronation of Haile Selassie I as King of Ethiopia. Rastafarians consider themselves to be the chosen people of God and are on earth to promote his power and peacefulness.

- Shinto: Shinto has no known founder or single sacred scripture. Shinto is wholly devoted to life in this world and emphasises man's essential goodness. Shinto does not split the universe into a natural physical world and a supernatural transcendent world. It regards everything as part of a single unified creation. Shinto also does not make the Western division between body and spirit – even spirit beings exist in the same world as human beings.

- Sikhism: Sikhism was founded in the Punjab by Guru Nanak and is a monotheistic religion. Sikhs think that religion should be practised by living in the world and coping with life's everyday problems. The Sikh ideal combines action and belief. To live a good life a person should do good deeds as well as meditating on God.
- Taoism: Taoism is an ancient tradition of philosophy and religious belief that is deeply rooted in Chinese customs and world view. Taoist ideas have become popular throughout the world through Tai Chi Chuan, Qigong and various martial arts.
- Unitarianism: Unitarianism is an open-minded and individualistic approach to religion that gives scope for a very wide range of beliefs and doubts. Unitarians are sceptical about any one person or tradition possessing the whole truth. They are also increasingly aware of the inherent value of diversity for the well-being of the natural world. With these points in mind, Unitarians suggest that human differences of opinion and lifestyle should be seen as potentially creative and enriching, rather than necessarily destructive.

It is important to note that religions have specific holy days. A multi-faith calendar is available at http://www.bbc.co.uk/religion/tools/calendar, which can enable work-based facilitators to develop awareness of students' specific religious needs during a work-based placement.

ACTIVITY 6.6

Are there aspects of your practice that would disadvantage a student religiously or spiritually?

What action could you take to address this?

What changes within your organisation would be needed? (This could be useful to include in your portfolio.)

Disability

The Disability Discrimination Act (1995) defines a disability as a physical or mental impairment that has a substantial and long-term adverse effect on a person's ability to carry out normal day-to-day activities. This was clarified in the Disability Discrimination Act 2005 (Department for Work and Pensions 2005) with the following points of clarification:

- substantial means neither minor nor trivial
- long-term means that the effect of the impairment has lasted or is likely to last for at least 12 months (there are special rules covering recurring or fluctuating conditions)
- normal day-to-day activities include everyday things like eating, washing, walking and going shopping
- a normal day-to-day activity must affect one of the 'capacities' listed in the Act which include mobility, manual dexterity, speech, hearing, seeing and memory.

Some conditions such as a tendency to set fires and hay fever are specifically excluded.

Provisions allow for people with a past disability to be covered by the scope of the Act. There are also additional provisions relating to people with progressive conditions. The Disability Discrimination Act (2005) amends the definition of disability, removing the requirement that a mental illness should be 'clinically well-recognised'.

People with HIV, cancer and multiple sclerosis will be deemed to be covered by the Disability Discrimination Act (2005) effectively from the point of diagnosis, rather than from the point when the condition has some adverse effect on their ability to carry out normal day-to-day activities.

It is important to note that a student may not have a disability, but cares for someone with a disability. The Carers (Equal Opportunities) Act 2004 ensures that carers are able to take up opportunities that people without caring responsibilities often take for granted, for example, working or studying or activities. The implications for work-based facilitators are that there may be a need to be aware of students' needs and make necessary adjustments.

ACTIVITY 6.7

Are there aspects of your practice that would disadvantage a student with a disability?

What action could you take to address this?

What changes organisationally would be needed to meet the needs of a student with a disability? (This could be useful to include in your portfolio.)

Sexuality and gender

The Government recognises the discrimination that many female, gay, lesbian and bisexual people face in today's society. The Employment Equality (Sexual Orientation) Regulations 2003 include an order to prohibit sexual orientation discrimination in the provision of goods, facilities and services, in education and in the execution of public functions.

Sex discrimination can take many forms and can impact upon people in different aspects of their life. The Equal Opportunities Commission (2010) asserts that women and men have the right not to be discriminated against because of their sex, in many aspects of their working life – from their recruitment and promotion prospects and how much they are paid, to all aspects of how they are treated by an employer and their colleagues, including when pregnant, and if they are dismissed.

Therefore, work-based facilitators need to ensure that students do not experience any discrimination on the basis of either gender or sexual orientation whilst on placement.

ACTIVITY 6.8

Are there aspects of your practice that would disadvantage a student due to their gender or sexual orientation?

What action could you take to address this?

What changes organisationally would be needed? (This could be useful to include in your portfolio.)

Age and generation

It is widely accepted that today's older people are in better health, live longer and independent lives, are better educated and have high expectations in terms of being useful and participating socially. Retirement is a new phase in life and for many people it represents an opportunity to do something completely different to their working life.

Access to learning and knowledge has much to offer to quality of life in older age. Research has highlighted that learning is good for older and retired people and has revealed that older people believe that learning helps to keep their brains active. Through the research, older people argued that learning stimulates their intellect and gives them pleasure and helps them to understand and cope with constant change in society. Some older people believe that the therapeutic value of learning is a way of ensuring good health.

Keeping active and involved in community helps maintain a sense of purpose and self-respect, particularly for those who have retired from paid work. It lessens the isolation felt by those cut off from social networks in the workplace and from their families and it has beneficial effects on physical and mental health.

Values can collide when members of different generations work and learn together. Having a better understanding of others can make the working and learning environment more productive. Work-based facilitators don't have to agree with the values of students coming from a different generation, but they should try to understand the mind-sets of different generations and how students approach the work placement as this will be based on their experiences. In addition, many students may provide a substantial amount of care for one or more elderly relatives. The Carers (Equal Opportunities) Act 2004 means that student carers need support in ensuring they have equity in placement experiences, with their role as a care provider acknowledged.

Work-based facilitators need to be aware of how they can support students from a range of diverse backgrounds to ensure that all students have an appropriate learning experience whilst on placement. The next part of this unit will introduce you to some strategies for ensuring equity in students' placement experience.

ACTIVITY 6.9

Are there aspects of your practice that would disadvantage a student due to their age?

What action could you take to address this?

What changes organisationally would be needed? (This could be useful to include in your portfolio.)

Strategies for supporting all students

ACTIVITY 6.10

Reflect on your teaching practice and one-to-one contact with students using the headings below. In what way do you think you could improve your communication skills?

- language
- written material
- your verbal communication
- your non-verbals
- your listening skills.

How could you incorporate these developments into your work with students? (This could be useful to include in your portfolio.)

People from diverse groups may encounter discrimination (unfair treatment) and prejudiced attitudes. Chouhan and Weaver (2012) state that the Government believes that race equality is essential to build strong, inclusive communities. There is a moral case for striving for race equality. It is a basic human right to be treated with equality and fairness. This is recognised in the European Convention on Human Rights and reflected in the Human Rights Act 1998. Furthermore, there is an economic case for (race) equality too, as everyone's potential can be utilised.

The Disability Discrimination Act 1995 gives people the right to ask for 'reasonable adjustments' to take account of their disability. For example, dyslexics can ask for more time in exams, or there can be agreement to use strategies that work for the individual whilst learning in the workplace.

In a facilitatory relationship, whether it is between two individuals or a group of people, communication and interaction provide the essential framework for the professional relationship to develop. It helps to build up trust and rapport, and it provides a process that is empowering, supportive and, when necessary, directive (Nadirshaw and Torry 2012). One of the principle barriers within a facilitatory relationship is the presence of 'professional power'. Power inequalities arise within facilitator and supervisee relationships, and between majority ethnic groups and minority ethnic groups.

Work-based facilitators should not only avoid discriminating against students but should help optimise student learning during a work-based placement. Many of the following recommendations constitute good practice that should be considered for all students as, under the Data Protection Act (1998), neither students nor the higher education institution are obliged to reveal the presence of a disability even if it disadvantages the student.

Davis (2008) believes that there are no universal solutions or specific rules for responding to ethnic, gender and cultural diversity in teaching, and that research on best practices is limited. Indeed, the topic is complicated, confusing and dynamic, and for some facilitators it is fraught with uneasiness, difficulty and discomfort. Perhaps the overriding principle is to be thoughtful and sensitive and do what you think is best. The section begins by looking at general ways of supporting students before looking at strategies that might be used for specific groups.

Communication

Communicating with others is an essential part of our everyday life. The need to communicate shows itself in many ways. It helps us establish relationships, share information and ideas, and give meanings to everything we do. Failure to give accurate and easily understood information can lead to anxiety (Mary Seacole Centre 2012). When we consider a social encounter, we may become aware of the many visible and invisible aspects of communication. The spoken word, the written message and the non-verbal gesture or facial expressions all play an important part in getting the message across. Similarly, these aspects are part of showing acknowledgement and understanding of the message. In effective communication, the shared meaning of the message is crucial to the outcome of the social encounter.

In cross-cultural encounters, the need to demonstrate effective communication assumes an even greater significance because there may be more scope for misunderstanding and conflicts. Thus, making the wrong assumptions about the cultural background of individuals and assuming that there is a specific way to interact with a person with a particular cultural background may lead to breakdown in communication, rendering it ineffective (Corey *et al.* 2011). However, work-based facilitators need to remember that people cannot be put into culturally specific boxes nor labelled by virtue of culture and race. Do not assume that the criteria for a certain cultural group are true for every student belonging to a particular disability, racial, ethnic, or cultural group.

There is relatively little agreement on where exactly the boundary between verbal and non-verbal communication may be drawn. Particularly, the importance of non-word utterances, such as a throat clearing noise, is highly debated. As with so many other cultural factors, non-verbal communication is subject to the interpretation of the non-verbal signs by the recipient of the message. Frequently, the interpretation and recognition of non-verbal messages is subconscious, and may therefore be extremely misleading in intercultural encounters TDKTutor (2012).

Power Learning (2012) highlights ways in which language can be used to avoid discrimination that is caused by placing one group of people below others, thus creating or perpetuating negative social stereotypes. Given the spirit of inclusivity in our culture, some suggestions are provided here to avoid derogatory language. The examples are by no means comprehensive, but serve to remind us of areas where language discrimination still exists and causes unnecessary misunderstandings in our daily communication with the general public. The spirit of the 'title' used to describe a person or group can be summed up by following six general principles:

- Don't single out a person's sex, race, ethnicity or other personal traits or characteristics (such as sexual orientation, age or a disability) when it has no direct bearing on the topic at hand. In other words, don't create or promote stereotype based on unavoidable human characteristics.

- Be consistent in your description of members of a group: Don't single out women to describe their physical beauty, clothes or accessories or note a disabled person's use of an aid, or refer to the race of the only minority in a group unless it is at that individual's request.
- Keep in mind that use of inclusive language is for general cases. Direct requests by individuals take precedence over general rules (e.g. Mr John Doe requests that his name is not used).
- Unless your writing is specifically focused on disabilities, avoid singling out one individual's disabilities simply for the sake of identification.
- Avoid using words that imply victimisation or create negative stereotypes. For example, don't use descriptors such as 'victim' or 'sufferer' for someone with a disease; just identify the disease. Avoid using words such as 'poor', 'unfortunate', or 'afflicted'.
- Don't say 'courageous' when you can say 'successful' or 'productive'.

Some general guidelines on not using gender-specific language include:

- Degender, don't regender (e.g., degender chairman to chair, don't regender it to chairwoman).
- Create gender-neutral terms: convert adjectives to nouns by adding -ist (e.g., active: activist).
- Replace occupational terms containing man and boy, if possible, with terms that include members of either gender.
- Avoid occupational designations having derogatory -ette and -ess endings.

Listening

It is also important that work-based facilitators listen to their students. Listening is divided into two main categories: passive and active. Passive listening is little more that hearing, whereas active listening involves listening with a purpose. This may be to gain information, obtain directions, understand others, solve problems, share interest, see how another person feels or show support. Clark (2010) identifies certain traits of active listeners:

- spend more time listening than talking
- do not finish the sentence of others
- do not answer questions with questions
- are aware of biases. We all have them... we need to control them
- never daydream or become preoccupied with their own thoughts when others talk
- let the other speaker talk. They do not dominate the conversation
- plan responses after the other person has finished speaking... NOT while they are speaking
- provide feedback, but do not interrupt incessantly
- analyse by looking at all the relevant factors and asking open-ended questions. Walk the person through their analysis (summarise)
- keep the conversation on what the speaker says... NOT on what interests them
- take brief notes. This forces them to concentrate on what is being said.

A number of authors identify certain key behaviours in effective non-verbal communication.

- Eye contact: Meyerson (2010) believes that looking directly at the person as you speak helps to communicate your sincerity and increases the directness of your message. It shows that you respect the person, which helps create a more positive relationship. Teachers who make eye contact open the flow of communication and convey interest, concern, warmth and credibility. However, according to TDKTutor (2012), people from some cultures may lower their gaze to convey respect, whereas this may be understood as insulting in other cultures. Direct eye contact may be seen as insulting in some cultures or convey attention in others.
- Facial expression: Ritts and Stein (2012) state that smiling is a powerful cue that transmits:
    - happiness
    - friendliness

- warmth
- liking
- affiliation.

Thus, work-based facilitators who smile frequently will be perceived as more likable, friendly, warm and approachable. Smiling is often contagious and students will react favourably and learn more.

- **Gestures**: failure to gesture while speaking will, according to Ritts and Stein (2012), result in a facilitator being perceived as boring, stiff and unanimated. A lively and animated teaching style captures students' attention, makes the material more interesting, facilitates learning and provides a bit of entertainment. Head nods, a form of gesture, communicate positive reinforcement to students and indicate that you are listening.
- **Distance**: the personal space, or the distance from other persons, is a powerful concept. Research suggests that it directly relates to our interpretation of the meaning of messages conveyed by the other person. For example, a person expressing anger is perceived as less threatening the further away that person is. However, if the person is close, the expression of anger becomes more threatening. In fact, physical closeness may itself be used to threaten the other person (TDKTutor 2012).

  Pay attention to how close you are to another person. Some people feel comfortable with physical closeness; others may be offended. Many cultures also place limitations on such closeness. You should look for signals of discomfort caused by invading students' space. Some of these are:
  - rocking
  - leg swinging
  - tapping
  - gaze aversion

  If you sense that someone feels uncomfortable, put a little more space between you and the other person(s) (Meyerson 2010).
- **Body position**: one way to be aware of cultural differences is to observe how people stand or sit while talking to others. Meyerson (2010) claims that you will be surprised how many people talk with their bodies turned away from those they're speaking to. Standing side by side may disconnect you from your partner, and standing face to face may seem confrontational. Instead, stand or sit at an angle from the other person. And, whenever possible, sit or stand at the same eye level as the other party, which signals that you're equals and decreases any feelings of intimidation. Speaking with your back turned or looking at the floor or ceiling should be avoided as it communicates disinterest (Clark 2010).
- **Touch**: although used most frequently during greetings and departures, touching may occur in a variety of circumstances, including during a conversation. Some cultures place great emphasis on physical contact between people during a conversation, while people from societies in which touching is limited may feel uncomfortable (TDKTutor 2012). Furthermore, the boundaries between the different levels of intimacy are somewhat blurred, even in one culture. However, across cultures, notions of acceptable touching behaviour may be completely different with the consequence that touching behaviour may frequently cause irritation and misinterpretation of what is intended with the touch.

Maun (2007) identifies the following behaviours as ones that should be avoided as they hinder effective communication:

- talking 'at' the other individual
- talking 'to' an individual
- talking 'about' an individual
- avoiding an individual or situation
- talking 'through' something or someone else.

ACTIVITY 6.11

To reflect on your non-verbal communication, agree with a student that you will video one of your meetings. On watching the video, identify the strengths and weaknesses in your non-verbal communication.

To further improve on your non-verbal communication, meet with a peer who will give you feed-back on your non-verbal communication.

List the action you should take to improve your non-verbal communication skills. (This could be useful to include in your portfolio.)

Student support strategies

Work-based facilitators may want to consider using some of the following strategies for support-ing specific groups of students.

Dyslexia

Bournemouth University (2012) states that individuals with dyslexia may not present with the same problem(s). Furthermore, the severity of a particular problem experienced by individuals may also vary. However, a number of possible strategies are outlined:

- Make learning outcomes and professional expectations clear.
- Provide clear instructions to the student.
- Keep a pocket book for notes.
- Note priorities and discuss notes with other students and staff.
- Repeat instructions to avoid misunderstanding.
- Write instructions in sequence.
- Jot notes on scrap paper and have them checked before committing them to paper.
- Double check for mistakes.
- Practise skills, before using them in 'normal' work situations under observation to ensure safe practice.

Disability

By agreeing to accept students on placement, the employer is providing a service to those students which, as such, will be included under Part 3 of the Disability Discrimination Act (1995) (Rights of Access: Goods Facilities and Services). The Act states that it is unlawful for a service provider to discriminate against a disabled person by:

- refusing to provide (or deliberately not providing) any service which it offers or provides to other students
- providing service of a lower standard or in a worse manner
- providing service on worse terms
- failing to comply with a duty to make reasonable adjustments if that failure has the effect of making it impossible or unreasonably difficult for the disabled person to make use of any such service.

The Department for Education and Skills (2002) provides some practical guidance on how to provide placements for disabled students. For example, have a written agreement with the placement provider, which outlines the responsibilities of the placement provider, the institution and students. Such an agreement might cover:

- physical access to the workplace
- responsibility for assessing the individual needs of disabled students
- who will pay (the institution or the placement provider) for any adjustments that need to be made for disabled students
- responsibilities for health and safety in the workplace
- procedures for risk assessment of activities associated with the work placement
- procedures for responding to any difficulties, including complaints and health emergencies
- procedures for providing feedback to the institution and the disabled student on the student's progress.

Further recommendations from the Department for Education and Skills (2002) cover preparing for a work-based placement. Primarily staff within the institution should meet with students and the work-based facilitator at an early stage to discuss students' support needs and what, if any, adjustments may need to be made. In many cases students may have a good idea of the types of support they need. Other students may not be aware of what equipment or support is available and might be useful in the unfamiliar work environment. Aspects which it might be relevant to cover in a discussion include:

- ensuring that students are appropriately prepared for placements – in some cases disabled students may need more preparation than other students
- ensuring access to work placements, including transport arrangements
- ensuring access to any equipment that the student may need to use on the work placement
- ensuring access to audio material and meetings for students with sensory impairments, including the use of interpreters, radio aids or subtitled videos
- ensuring access to visual material and documents for students with visual impairments or dyslexia, including providing printed materials in accessible formats or providing material on tape
- ensuring access to complex instructions for students with learning difficulties
- ensuring that placements are appropriate for students with mental health problems or who experience fatigue, etc. In some cases a balance may need to be struck between allowing students access to the widest range of placement opportunity and consideration of the demands involved
- clarifying arrangements for support workers who may accompany students, e.g. sign language interpreters, personal assistants, etc.
- ensuring ongoing support for those students who may need it through visits or telephone calls, particularly at the start of the placement.

Finally, the Department for Education and Skills (2002) also recommends use of a checklist, which can guide work-based facilitators to assess the suitability of their workplace for disabled students:

- Is there an agreement between the institution, placement provider and student about what adjustments are required, and who will provide them?
- Does the placement organiser keep in constant touch with students and placement providers to ensure that necessary adjustments are made to make the placement physically accessible for those with sensory and mobility impairments?
- Is the placement physically accessible for those with sensory and mobility impairments?
- Where physical access is not possible, have arrangements been made to relocate important meetings, etc?
- Do students have access to suitable methods of transport if required?
- Will communication in the workplace be accessible to those with sensory impairments?
- When a student is unable to attend regularly, have alternative arrangements been made to enable the student to continue with his/her placement?
- Are there clear written guidelines about providing access to work placements?

Work-based facilitators should assess the needs of the student in work-related learning situations. FERL (2003a) believes that it would be useful to address the following questions:

- Has the learner undertaken work placements before?
- What is their employment history?
- What were the issues and solutions in previous employment?
- What (assistive) equipment does the learner have and how portable is it?
- Will the learner require the installation of specific software on a computer, e.g. screen-reading software?

Assessment, as previously discussed in Unit 5, forms an important part of a work-based placement, even if it is only a formative assessment. Disabled students may require additional help to ensure equity with other students when undertaking a work-based assessment. It is important to evaluate exactly what is being assessed and to ensure that whatever is being assessed will not be made more difficult by the presence of impairment. In an assessed work-based practical situation, a learner with dexterity problems should not be penalised for not being able to measure out quantities of a chemical substance, when they can instruct a support worker precisely how to do this. In this way the learner has demonstrated equivalent knowledge to his or her non-disabled peers.

In many cases learners will not need to undertake an alternative exercise, but may need additional time to undertake the task or to use assistive technology or additional human support or a combination of both.

FERL (2003b) set out some important considerations, such as:

- What learning outcomes are to be assessed? For example, is spelling, grammar and correct syntax a criterion for the assessment – if not, will the learner be penalised for bad grammar? Is the learner being assessed on their knowledge and skill, rather than aspects of their impairment?
- Can the learner do all elements of a task? If not, what adjustments can be made so that the learner can demonstrate his or her skills and knowledge? For example, in an assessment where the aim is to create an advertising poster, could, for example, a blind learner submit a radio jingle instead?
- Are there any implications for marking? For example, how will a tutor assess an oral presentation given in British Sign Language, when it is important to assess the learner, not the skill of the interpreter?
- Will the learner be able to demonstrate their skills and knowledge equally to their non-disabled peers? Have these alternatives been explored with the learner and are they confident in the validity and equanimity of the assessment process?

Carers

Many students may have responsibility to provide care for another person (or persons), often because this person has a disability. Directgov (2012b) states that help from your employer, which may reasonably be applied to students undertaking a work-based placement, could include:

- access to a telephone so that you can call the person you are caring for
- a reserved car-parking space, to make getting in and out of work quicker and easier
- reasonable notice if overtime or working from home is necessary.

ACTIVITY 6.12

As a result of reading this unit, reflect on what areas you think you need to address to develop your own practice in meeting diverse student needs.

What action could you take to do this? (This could be useful to include in your portfolio.)

Conclusion

It is important to remember that students bring different talents and styles of learning to work-based placements. Brilliant students in the seminar room may be all thumbs in the lab or art studio. Students rich in hands-on experience may not do so well with theory. Students need the opportunity to show their talents and learn in ways that work for them. Then they can be pushed to learn in new ways that do not come so easily (Chickering and Gamson 2012). The role of the work-based facilitator is to ensure that no students are disadvantaged or discriminated against, but are treated equitably to ensure optimum student learning.

References

BBC (2012) Religions. www.bbc.co.uk/religion/religions.

Bournemouth University (2012) *Supporting Students with Dyslexia.* http://www.bournemouth.ac.uk/disability_support/staff/dyslexia.html

Carers (Equal Opportunities) Act (2004) www.legislation.gov.uk/ukpga/2004/15/contents

Cliffs Notes (2012) *Race and Ethnicity Defined.* www.cliffsnotes.com/study_guide/Race-and-Ethnicity-Defined.topicArticleId-26957,articleId-26884.html

Clark, D. (2010) *Communication and Leadership.* www.nwlink.com/%7Edonclark/leader/leadcom.html

Chickering, A. W. and Gamson, Z. F. (2012) *Seven Principles for Good Practice in Undergraduate Education.* http://honolulu.hawaii.edu/intranet/committees/FacDevCom/guidebk/teachtip/7princip.htm

Chouhan, K. and Weaver, D. (2012) *Transcultural Communication and Health Care Practice: Race equality management.* www.rcn.org.uk/resources/transcultural/raceequalitymanagement/index.php

Corey, G., Schneider Corey, M. and Callanan, P. (2011) *Issues and Ethics in the Helping Professions*, 8th edn. Brooks Cole.

Culley, L., Hudson, N. and Van Rooij, F. (2009) *Marginalized Reproduction.* Earthspan.

Data Protection Act (1998) www.legislation.gov.uk/ukpga/1998/29/contents

Davis, B. G. (2008) *Diversity and Complexity in the Classroom.* http://ets.tlt.psu.edu/learningdesign/audience/diversestudents

Department for Education and Skills (2002) *Providing Work Placements for Disabled Students.* www.lifelonglearning.co.uk/placements/placeme1.pdf

Department for Work and Pensions (2005) Disability Discrimination Act (2005) www.legislation.gov.uk/ukpga/2005/13/contents

Directgov (2012a) *Age Discrimination.* www.direct.gov.uk/en/Employment/ResolvingWorkplaceDisputes/DiscriminationAtWork/DG_10026429

Directgov (2012b) *Caring for Someone.* www.direct.gov.uk/CaringForSomeone/CarersAndEmployment/CarersAndEmploymentArticles/fs/en?CONTENT_ID=4000206&chk=H10zrD

Disability Discrimination Act (1995) www.legislation.gov.uk/ukpga/1995/50/contents

Disability Discrimination (Northern Ireland) Order (2006) www.ofmdfmni.gov.uk/index/equality/disability/new-disability-discrimination-order.htm

Employment Equality (Sexual Orientation) Regulations (2003) www.opsi.gov.uk/si/si2003/20031661.htm

Equal Opportunities Commission (2010) *Your Rights at Work.* www.equalityhumanrights.com/advice-and-guidance/your-rights/gender/sex-discrimination-your-rights-at-work

Equality Act (2010) www.legislation.gov.uk/ukpga/2010/15/contents

Fernandez, V. M. and Fernandez, K. M. (2012) *Transcultural Nursing: Basic Concepts and Case Studies.* www.culturediversity.org/index.html

European Court of Human Rights (2010) *The European Convention on Human Rights.* www.echr.coe.int/ECHR/EN/Header/Basic+Texts/The+Convention+and+additional+protocols/The+European+Convention+on+Human+Rights

FERL (2003a) *Work Experience and Work-related Learning.* www.excellencegateway.org.uk/page.aspx?o=149435

FERL (2003b) *Alternative Assessment.* www.excellencegateway.org.uk/page.aspx?o=149399

Geiger, J. N. and Davidhizar, R. E. (2008) *Transcultural Nursing. Assessment and Intervention*, 8th edn. Mosby Elsevier.

Hofstede, G., Minkov, M. and Gert, J. (2010) *Cultures and Organizations: Software of the Mind.* McGraw-Hill.

Honolulu Community College (2012) *Culturally Effective Communication.* http://honolulu.hawaii.edu/intranet/committees/FacDevCom/guidebk/teachtip/culture1.htm

Human Rights Act (1998) www.legislation.gov.uk/ukpga/1998/42/contents

Mary Seacole Centre (2012) *The MELTING Pot Project Web Site.* www.maryseacole.com/maryseacole/melting/validated.asp

Maun, C. (2007) *Conflict Management: What Really Works? Here's Proven Solutions.* www.clintmaun.com/index.php5?cID=283

Meyerson, H. (2010) *Honing your Nonverbal Communication Skills.* www.confidencecenter.com/art11.htm

Mitchell, J. (2012) *Understanding Dyslexia.* www.understandingdyslexia.co.uk

Nadirshaw, Z. and Torry, B. (2012) *Transcultural Health Care Practice: Transcultural Clinical Supervision in Health Care Practice.* www.rcn.org.uk/resources/transcultural/clinicalsupervision/index.php

Power Learning (2012) *Dos and Don't's of Inclusive Language.* http://blog.powerlearning21.com/2011/01/dos-and-donts-of-inclusive-language

Purnell, L. D. and Paulanka, B. J. (2008) *Transcultural Health Care. A Culturally Competent Approach,* 3rd ed. F A Davis Company.

Ritts, V. and Stein, J. R. (2012) *Six Ways to Improve Your Nonverbal Communication.* http://honolulu.hawaii.edu/intranet/committees/FacDevCom/guidebk/teachtip/commun-1.htm

Royal College of Nursing (2006a) *Diversity Appraisal Resource Guide.* www.rcn.org.uk/publications/pdf/diversity-appraisal.pdf

Royal College of Nursing (2006b) *Transcultural Health Care Practice: An Educational Resource for Nurses and Health Care Practitioners.* www.rcn.org.uk/resources/transcultural/index.php

TDKTutor (2012) *Non-verbal Communication.* http://tkdtutor.com/TOPICS/Self-Defense/Non-Verbal-Information/Non-Verbal-Information-02.htm

Portfolio completion guidelines

Many accrediting bodies and or higher education providers will have specific requirements for completing a portfolio. We recommend that you find out what these requirements are before starting to produce your portfolio.

The main purpose of this guide, based upon the work of Leith and Mulholland (2000), is to present information on the process and procedure involved in developing a portfolio which might be a requirement for the assessment of the toolkit. Contact your nearest accrediting body to get further details.

Claiming credit for prior experiential learning

One method of claiming credit for your learning is the process of claiming accreditation for prior (experiential) learning (AP(E)L). The first thing you have to come to terms with is that claiming credit through the AP(E)L process is very different from the traditional process of higher education.

The traditional method involves enrolling on taught courses where the content of the course and the nature of the assessment is determined by academic staff.

With AP(E)L, you are primarily responsible for determining whether or not you have achieved the learning outcomes required for the module and how best you can demonstrate that achievement.

Claiming specific credit

You will be claiming that the learning you have achieved through experience is equivalent to that required to meet the learning outcomes of a specified module/modules on the professional development programme.

This process is competed in two stages:

1 Drawing up an AP(E)L proposal for approval.
2 Preparing a claim for specific credit, which will include a portfolio of evidence and reflective account of learning.

The development of a portfolio will be required for both AP(E)L and the more traditional assessment of learning.

On completing this process you should have:

- identified experience/s relevant to module learning outcomes
- analysed and systematically reflected upon these experiences
- identified and provided evidence of significant learning achievement from experience in terms of:

○   knowledge gained
○   skills and competencies acquired
○   attitudes changed/formulated
- compiled the evidence in a portfolio to support a claim for credit.

Stage 1: Preparation and submission of a portfolio

Step 1 – Identifying module learning outcomes

These will be found in the relevant accrediting bodies' documents and will constitute the framework to which you will match your own learning.

Step 2 – Identifying relevant experience

Relevant and credible learning may have resulted from:

- employment
- education and training activities (e.g. short courses, workshops, seminars, personal reading)
- leisure-time activities and interests
- personal experience (such as parenting and voluntary work).

Your task here is to list experience/s from your past which will relate specifically to the learning outcomes identified in Step 1.

Step 3 – Analysing and reflecting on that experience

This is necessary in order to specify learning achieved that is equivalent to the level of knowledge and understanding that is required to meet the module learning outcomes.

This part of the process relates particularly to the academic level of your learning. It will require further reading in order to consolidate your knowledge and understanding of the subject area and will form the basis of your reflective account of learning.

You will need to undertake this process for each of the learning outcomes.

Step 4 – Writing a clear statement of the learning identified

For each of the learning outcomes you will need to be able to list what you know and are able to do in order to meet the learning outcomes.

You may find it helpful to summarise this process in the form of a table and matrix in which you note the *knowledge and understanding*, *skills and competencies* and *attitudes and values* distilled from your experience that relate to each of the outcomes. (See the introductory chapter of the toolkit.)

Step 5 – Identifying the type of evidence

Which evidence would confirm that the learning identified has been met? In identifying appropriate evidence, you should bear the following points in mind:

- Not all evidence will come from one source. Most of your evidence will come from your work, but you should consider other evidence from voluntary work or other activities.
- A single piece of evidence may be relevant to more than one learning outcome.

Nature of evidence

Evidence can be *direct* or *indirect*. Direct evidence reflects *your own work*. Examples might include:

- action plans – objectives and results
- budget or financial forecasts
- monthly or annual reports
- selected extracts from work diaries
- articles/books you have written or to which you have contributed
- a training plan you have devised
- procedures for which you have been responsible.

Indirect evidence is information from others *about you*. Examples might include:

- statements from employers/customers/clients
- supporting letters from managers
- newspaper articles about you.

Generally speaking, direct evidence is stronger and, for that reason, is preferable to indirect evidence.

Step 6 – Drawing up the proposal

The proposal specifies the learning for which credit is sought and the type of evidence that you will produce to support your claim for specific credit. It will also define the advice/guidance you require to complete the process and the times when this will occur. This will be specified in the learning agreement.

This learning agreement will be drawn up in consultation with your Advisor and will include:

- details of supervision arrangements, if any
- the submission date for your claim for specific credit.

(In order to submit a portfolio, you will have to compile your portfolio of evidence and write a reflective account of your learning. This process is dealt with in Stage 2, which is detailed below.)

Step 7 – Completing the relevant forms and submitting your proposal

The statement of learning outcomes, list of evidence and the learning agreement should be submitted via your Advisor by the agreed date.

Step 8 – Consideration of the proposal by the course team

Step 9 – Approval (or otherwise) of the proposal

The result of the Board's consideration will be communicated to you in writing.

Step 10 – Register for the appropriate module and pay the required fee

Stage 2: Preparing a portfolio

By this stage you have received approval of your proposal. The final stage involves compiling your portfolio of evidence, writing a reflective account of your learning and submitting your portfolio.

Compiling a portfolio of evidence

In compiling the evidence of your learning the following steps are suggested:

Step 1 – Making an outline plan of your portfolio

This should consist of:

- a contents list
- a brief introduction
- a statement of the learning claimed
- a package of appropriate and valid evidence that supports the learning claimed.

Step 2 – Collating and itemising the evidence

Decide what evidence to include. The main aims are:

- to show evidence of all the learning outcomes; and
- to present your achievements as effectively as possibly.

Look at the material you have got and *be selective* – choose concise, clear samples of your work. This is much more valuable to an assessor than large amounts of material which need to be sifted through to 'find' the learning. When selecting items, it may be helpful to ask yourself:

- How does this item help to prove my learning?
- Is it the best evidence for this learning outcome?
- Is it sufficient – or do I need more?

Other issues to consider are discussed below.

Confidentiality

The need for confidentiality may result in some materials you wish to use not being available for reproduction. You may deal with this problem in several ways, for example:

- If you are offering evidence for counselling, you could ask your clients/students for permission to use information related to them.
- If you are presenting a confidential report or reflective diary, you could delete information that identifies individuals or institutions.
- If you are uncertain, check with your manager or Advisor before including the evidence.

Availability

Sometimes you may have learning for which there is no readily available evidence. You should discuss this with your Advisor, who may be able to suggest an alternative way of demonstrating your achievement. If you know you have the learning, do not be discouraged from including it because it is difficult to evidence.

Authenticity

You need to clearly demonstrate to the assessors that the evidence you submit *verifies your learning*. Thus, if you are including work that you have contributed to along with others, you need to identify the work that was *exclusively yours*. Your reflective account of learning may be helpful with this.

Cross-referencing

Often one item of evidence will relate to several learning outcomes. Consequently, the assessor needs to be clearly directed to the appropriate area. A clearly constructed portfolio and good referencing are important.

Currency

With a portfolio, assessors are looking for evidence that supports your current level of skill and knowledge, rather than something you could do in the past. For example, a certificate showing that you completed a counselling course four years ago may also be supported by evidence that you are still using those counselling skills.

Step 3 – Writing the contents of the portfolio

While there is no set format for this, it is suggested that you use the learning outcomes as section headings.

You should clearly demonstrate how each piece of evidence relates to each learning outcome. Documentation that constitutes evidence is usually written for a different audience, so it is helpful to provide some degrees of explanation and/or comment with it.

Step 4 – Preparing the portfolio for submission

The aim should be to present your portfolio in a way that is helpful to someone who is seeking evidence of your learning:

- Where appropriate, contents should be typewritten.
- Evidence should be contained in a ring-binder file.
- Avoid including loose pieces of paper or separate documents, as these may get separated from your main portfolio.
- You are advised to make a copy of your portfolio and retain it for future reference.

Writing a reflective account of learning

The purpose of this aspect of the process is to relate your prior experiential learning to the academic content of the module for which you are claiming credit.

The aim is to demonstrate that you have an adequate knowledge and understanding of the subject area that has been learned through experience rather than study.

You will be advised to do some further reading in order to consolidate your knowledge and understanding of the subject in which your prior learning is located. A useful starting point is the reading list provided for the appropriate module.

General guidelines

Your reflective account of learning should be a focused piece of writing that puts the learning you have achieved into context. In relation to specific learning outcomes, you should aim to communicate fully and effectively how your learning has developed, drawing on and referring to supporting evidence from your portfolio and reading that you have done.

The first and most important aspect is how you reflect on development of your learning. Although many professional skills are best assessed and validated by demonstration, learning goes much further than doing. You do not just learn how to do things, you learn attitudes and values about what you are doing. You understand why a procedure is important to help you recognise that academic work involves analysis and critical thinking to a greater degree than in many work places or life experiences. In this context you might wish to use critical incident analysis to help you reflect on how particular experiences helped you learn.

There is no set format for the reflective account of the learning. You may wish to use the learning outcomes of the module for which you are claiming credit as a basis but, however you structure your account, it should:

- demonstrate your ability to reflect on your experience and extract from it appropriate learning
- be relevant to the specified learning outcomes
- refer directly to supporting evidence
- show understanding of the relevant academic theory, referring to particular reading where appropriate
- provide a contextual framework for your claim, showing clearly how you came to achieve your learning. In this instance it may be helpful to think of the reflective account as the 'story' of your learning, focusing on specific learning outcomes and showing how the evidence that you have included supports these.

A bibliography of texts consulted must be attached to your reflective account of learning. Your AP(E)L Adviser will provide guidance on the appropriate format for this. Your reflective account of learning should be limited to 2,500 words.

Critical incident analyses

What constitutes a critical incident? It is:

- an incident in which you feel your intervention/involvement really made a difference either directly or indirectly
- an incident that went unusually well
- an incident that did not go as planned
- an incident that is very ordinary and typical
- an incident that you feel captures the learning outcomes to be met
- an incident that was particularly demanding.

What to include in your description of a critical incident:

- the context of the incident, where it happened in relation to your work/life experience
- a detailed description of what happened
- why the incident is critical to you and the learning outcome/s under consideration
- what competence and performance were criteria involved
- your analyses, reflection and evaluation of what took place
- what evidence is available to support your discussion
- who can verify your account, competence and evidence.

The assessment process

The portfolio and reflective account of learning may be forwarded to two appropriate academic assessors. The assessors will independently assess the evidence of learning against the module learning outcomes, using the following criteria:

- Validity – evidence submitted should be appropriate to the learning claimed.
- Reliability – the context to which there is inter-assessor agreement or consistency.
- Sufficiency – the quality and range of evidence should be sufficient to demonstrate competence across the full range of learning outcomes for the placement.
- Authenticity – the evidence must be verifiable.
- Currency – concerns the 'regency' of the evidence.
- Level – the standard of achievement reached on completion of the learning outcomes of a specific module.

Following external moderation of assessment of the portfolio of evidence and reflective account of learning a recommendation will be forwarded to the Board of Examiners that credit (the award) be made (or not).

Reference

Leith, H. and Mulholland, J. (2000) *Preparing a Claim for Specific Credit*. University of Ulster.

Index

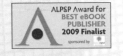